Preparing Your Doctoral Capstone

This practical and informative workbook guides occupational therapy doctorate students through every step of the capstone project and experience.

The workbook acknowledges the variability in capstone requirements and supports students by providing strategies to address common components. Each chapter offers tips and advice on topics such as identifying a need, finding a mentor and experiential site, conducting a literature review, developing project objectives, developing experiential objectives, and dissemination of the outcomes. Guiding students to develop a meaningful and productive capstone project and experience, the book includes worksheets and samples of completed student projects and experiences at each stage of the process.

This is the ideal guide for any occupational therapy doctorate student aiming to undertake a successful capstone project, as well as the perfect complement for Doctoral Capstone Coordinators (DCC) and didactic classroom teaching and learning.

Pamela A. Kasyan-Howe, a DCC with over 20 years in higher education, has developed curriculum for associate to doctoral programs. She has held roles as program director, academic fieldwork coordinator, and doctoral coordinator. Pamela has served as an AOTA doctoral mentor, Chair of FLOTEC, and FOTA SIS Chair for Fieldwork and Capstone Education. She has published and presented at state, national, and international venues on fieldwork, doctoral capstone, ethics, and leadership.

Kristin Domville is a DCC at the University of St. Augustine for Health Sciences, Miami campus. Her extensive experience in clinical practice and academic leadership underscores her commitment to advancing the field of occupational therapy and mentoring the next generation of OT practitioners.

Michael A. Pizzi developed one of NY's first OTD programs and is a former DCC. He received the Award for Excellence in the Advancement of Occupational Therapy and became one of the youngest Fellows of the American Occupational Therapy Foundation, given to those who demonstrate scholarship, leadership, and service. Dr. Pizzi was guest editor for *AJOT* special issues on HIV/AIDS, childhood obesity, and health, well-being, and quality of life, and created the Pizzi Health and Wellness Assessment.

'*Preparing Your Doctoral Capstone* is an invaluable resource for occupational therapy students and doctoral capstone coordinators. It provides a comprehensive guide through the capstone project and experience, from inception to dissemination, with a distinct emphasis on the workbook nature of the book. The inclusion of activities and worksheets in each chapter fosters critical thinking and clarifies each stage of project development. This workbook stands out for its practical approach, helping students create, disseminate, and sustain meaningful projects as well as identify and develop impactful capstone experiences. It's a must-have for anyone involved in occupational therapy programs.'

Karen Jacobs, OT, EdD, OTR, CPE, FAOTA, *past AOTA president*

'*Preparing Your Doctoral Capstone* offers a fantastic overview and insights into best practices for developing a capstone project and capstone experience. Offering options for stages of capstone development, the workbook can align with different curriculum designs but also provide specific guidance to create individual, rigorous capstones. It is an essential resource for doctoral coordinators and occupational therapy doctorate students.'

Barbara L. Kornblau, JD, OTR/L, FAOTA, DASPE, CCM, CDMS, *past AOTA president*

'Offering a superb overview and insightful best practices, *Preparing Your Doctoral Capstone* is an invaluable, exquisitely structured guide for developing a capstone project and experience. The workbook uses an engaging narrative style and an iterative approach that captures the reader's attention while scaffolding learning. Each chapter contains activities that guide learners to apply multiple concepts and provides samples of those applications. Descriptions, underlying evidence and rationale for each stage of capstone development, as well as FAQ's, are presented throughout. Efforts have been made to ensure compatibility with various curriculum designs while delivering rigorous, structured guidance for individual capstones. This text is destined to be an essential tool for doctoral coordinators and occupational therapy doctorate students.'

Ellen L. Kolodner, MSS,OTR, FAOTA, *President, OT Leaders and Legacies Society and recipient of the AOTA Award of Merit*

Preparing Your Doctoral Capstone

A Workbook for Occupational Therapy Students

Pamela A. Kasyan-Howe, Kristin Domville, and Michael A. Pizzi

Routledge
Taylor & Francis Group

NEW YORK AND LONDON

Designed cover image: Getty Images

First published 2025
by Routledge
605 Third Avenue, New York, NY 10158

and by Routledge
4 Park Square, Milton Park, Abingdon, Oxon, OX14 4RN

Routledge is an imprint of the Taylor & Francis Group, an informa business

© 2025 Pamela A. Kasyan-Howe, Kristin Domville, and Michael A. Pizzi.

The right of Pamela A. Kasyan-Howe, Kristin Domville, and Michael A. Pizzi to be identified as authors of this work has been asserted in accordance with sections 77 and 78 of the Copyright, Designs and Patents Act 1988.

Library of Congress Cataloging-in-Publication Data
Names: Kasyan-Howe, Pamela A., author. | Domville, Kristin, author. |
  Pizzi, Michael, author.
Title: Preparing your doctoral capstone : a workbook for occupational therapy
  students / Pamela A. Kasyan-Howe, Kristin Domville, and Michael A. Pizzi.
Description: Abindon, Oxon ; New York, NY : Routledge, 2025. | Includes
  bibliographical references and index.
Identifiers: LCCN 2024042435 | ISBN 9781032897271 (hardback) | ISBN
  9781638221029 (paperback) | ISBN 9781003525868 (ebook)
Subjects: LCSH: Occupational therapy—Study and teaching (Graduate)
Classification: LCC RM735.42 .K37 2025 | DDC 615.8/515072—dc23/
  eng/20241223
LC record available at https://lccn.loc.gov/2024042435

ISBN: 978-1-032-89727-1 (hbk)
ISBN: 978-1-63822-102-9 (pbk)
ISBN: 978-1-003-52586-8 (ebk)

DOI: 10.4324/9781003525868

Typeset in Frutiger LT Pro
by Apex CoVantage, LLC

Access the Support Material: www.routledge.com/9781638221029

Dedication

I owe a special gratitude to my husband, James Howe, for his boundless patience and unwavering support of our family and all my endeavors. To my children, Jacob, Aiden, Chase, and Teagan, for their grace and silent sacrifices for the times I couldn't be with them. Finally, for my parents, Linda and George Kasyan for giving me a love of learning and whose unwavering encouragement and love fueled my passion for occupational therapy and education, I am deeply grateful.

– Pamela A. Kasyan-Howe

This workbook is dedicated to all occupational therapy students who strive for excellence in the profession of OT. May this resource empower you to achieve your highest potential and make a lasting impact within the profession of OT. To my husband Mark, whose unwavering encouragement and love have fueled my passion for occupational therapy and education. Lastly, to my precious daughter Giavanna, your sweet laughter, smile, and boundless energy provided me with the motivation to keep writing.

– Kristin Domville

I have been an OT since 1981, when a bachelor degree was required as entry level. I have witnessed the evolution and progression of the profession on many levels, especially in education. The OTD provides students (facilitated by doctoral coordinators and faculty) opportunities to develop projects that are meaningful and satisfying to them, often on a personal basis; opportunities that contribute to improving society and communities. Those projects also promote the profession in ways that are immeasurable. So, I dedicate this workbook to those innovative and creative students who intend to change the world.

– Michael A. Pizzi

Contents

Figures

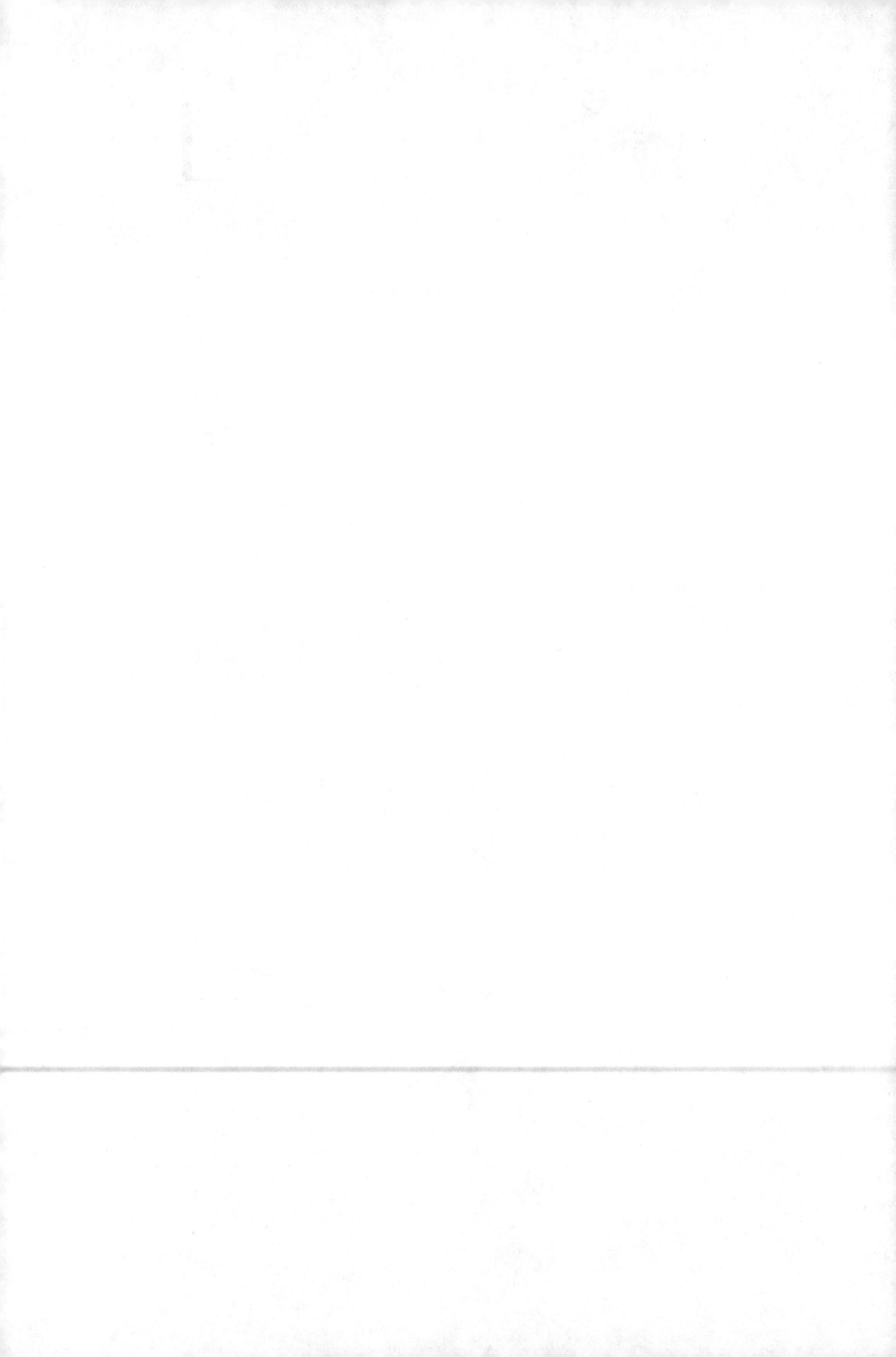

Tables

Worksheets

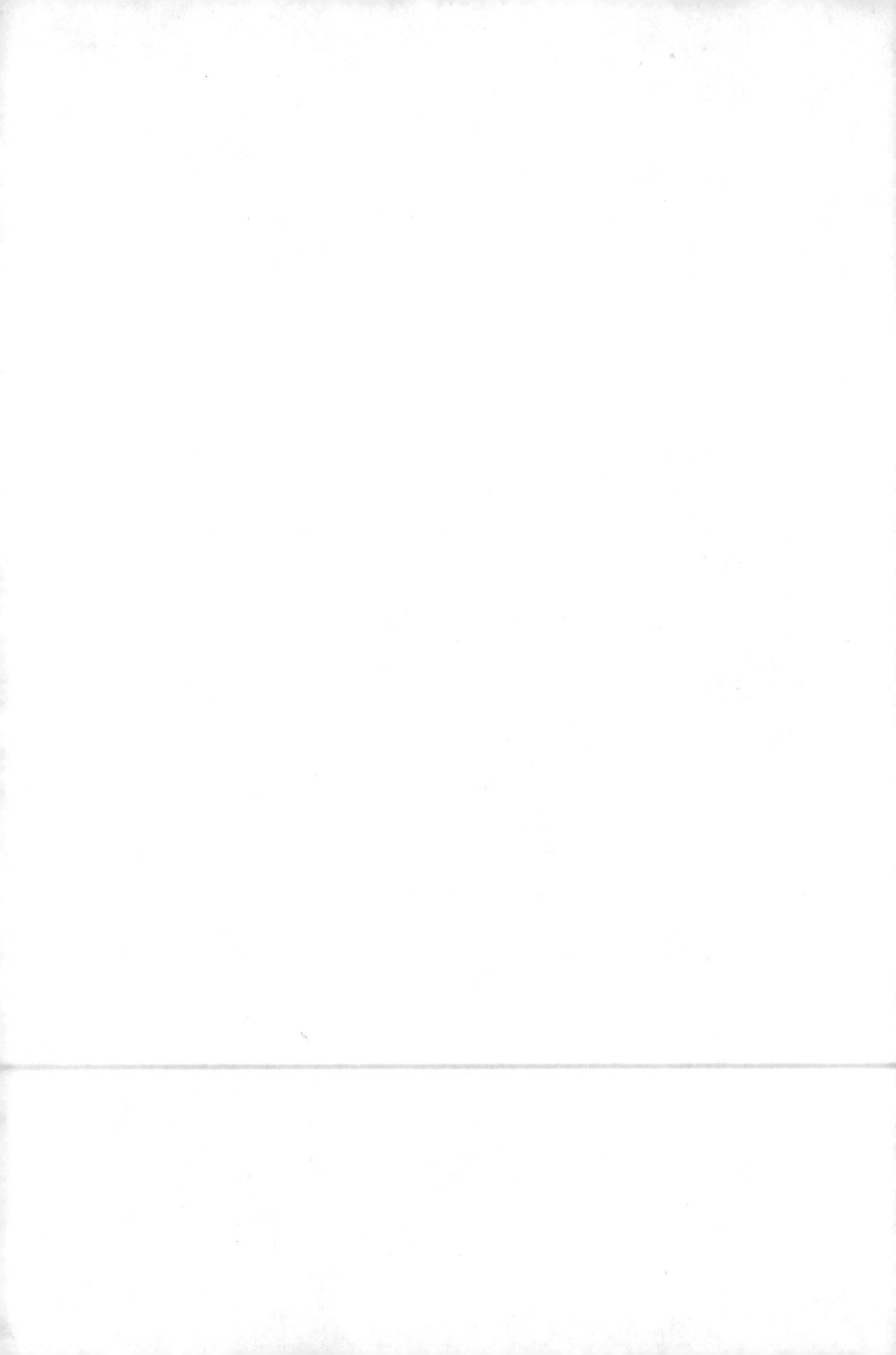

Learning Activities

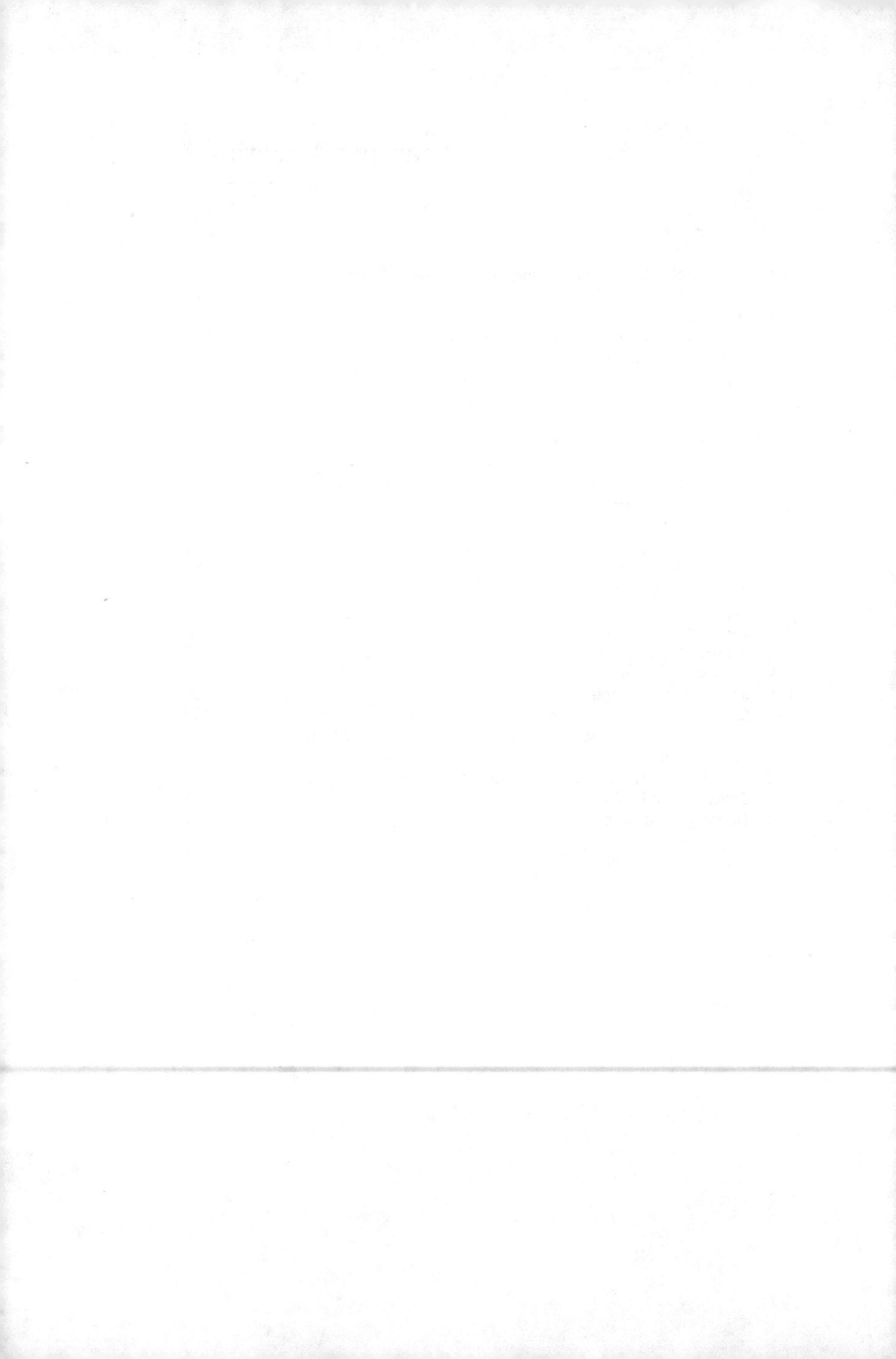

About the Authors

Pamela A. Kasyan-Howe is a Doctoral Capstone Coordinator at the University of St. Augustine for Health Sciences, Miami campus. Her research focus is on marginalized populations, student learning, education and ethics, policy and public administration. Over the course of her career, she has gained clinical experience in TBI, SCI, neuro, movement disorders, dementia, acute care, work hardening, orthopedics, upper quadrant rehabilitation, and hand therapy. Dr. Kasyan-Howe has demonstrated her passion for higher education and student experiential learning for over 20 years. She developed curriculum for associates, master's, and doctoral level programs. She has served as AOTA Doctoral Capstone Coordinator mentor, Chairperson of Florida Occupational Therapy Educational Consortium (FLOTEC), and Florida Occupational Therapy Association (FOTA) SIS Chair for Fieldwork and Capstone Education. She has published and presented at state, national, and international venues on fieldwork, doctoral capstone, ethics, and leadership. She has mentored over 50 student presentations at state and national venues.

Kristin Domville, PhD, DrOT, OTR/L, brings 18 years of diverse experience in occupational therapy, specializing in neurorehabilitation, mental health, physical disabilities, and education. Her career includes eight years as the OTA program director, demonstrating her leadership and commitment to education. Currently, she is the Doctoral Capstone Coordinator at the University of St. Augustine for Health Sciences, Miami campus, where she guides students in the doctoral capstone process.

Dr. Domville's research interests encompass academic advising, occupational therapy in mental health, and OT leadership. She is an active contributor to the professional community, having presented at national and state conferences on topics related to advancing occupational therapy practice, particularly in physical disabilities and education, with a focus on the doctoral capstone.

In addition to her academic and clinical roles, Dr. Domville serves as the Special Interest Chair for Physical Disabilities in the Florida Occupational Therapy Association (FOTA), where she advocates for best practices and innovations in the OT profession. Her extensive experience and dedication to occupational therapy make her a valuable mentor and leader, committed to advancing the profession and supporting the development of future occupational therapists.

Michael A. Pizzi, PhD, OTR/L, FAOTA helped create one of the first OTD programs in NY and is a former Doctoral Capstone Coordinator. Dr. Pizzi is a recipient of the Award for Excellence in the Advancement of Occupational Therapy and was one of the youngest therapists to become a Fellow of the American Occupational Therapy Foundation (FAOTA), given to those who demonstrate scholarship, leadership, and service to the profession. He was guest editor for *AJOT* special issues on HIV/AIDS, childhood obesity, and health, well-being and quality of life. Dr. Pizzi created the Pizzi Health and Wellness Assessment (PHWA) and the Pizzi Healthy Weight Management Assessment (PHWMA), both of which are used internationally. He has published over 70 peer-reviewed journal articles and chapters in textbooks on topics including HIV rehabilitation, hospice, entrepreneurship, childhood obesity and health, well-being and quality of life, and was a forerunner in these areas. There are over 100 lectures, workshops, and keynote addresses focusing on advancing occupational therapy practice in the area of health and well-being to his credit. Dr. Pizzi is co-editor of the textbook *Interprofessional Perspectives for Community Practice: Promoting Health, Well-Being and Quality of Life*.

Acknowledgements

The authors acknowledge Dr. Lisa Bagby, author of the chapter on needs assessment, whose collegiality, diligence, and writing contribute greatly to this workbook. We also acknowledge the diligence with which the team at Routledge, particularly Russell George and Amy Thomson, helped make this workbook a reality.

(PKH) I acknowledge all occupational therapy students and practitioners who work to improve society through participation in occupation. A special acknowledgment goes to my mentors and colleagues, whose guidance and support have been invaluable throughout my career – specifically Barbara Kornblau, for her lifetime of friendship, leadership, and mentorship. For my co-authors, Kristin Domville for her dedication to a pursuit of rigorous student outcomes, and Michael A. Pizzi for his prodding, feedback and guidance, and lifetime of service to our wonderful profession.

(KD) I extend my heartfelt gratitude to my co-authors, Pamela Kasyan-Howe and Michael A. Pizzi, for their invaluable contributions and collaboration on this workbook. Your expertise and dedication have been instrumental in its creation. I am grateful to my mentor Dr. Lawrence Faulkner who has left me with his invaluable guidance, inspiration, and knowledge. A special acknowledgment to my academic colleagues and OT students.

(MP) Michael A. Pizzi wishes to acknowledge his co-authors Pamela Kasyan-Howe and Kristin Domville for their collaboration on this important text. He also acknowledges the academic colleagues and students who helped his critical thinking about the OTD which led to developing strategies to ever improve the OTD capstone.

Introduction to Your Doctoral Work and This Workbook

When you chose to engage in doctoral work, whether entry level or post-professional, you no doubt had a reason for doing so. Some people want more knowledge, or more expertise in a specific area, while others intend to teach at some point and know that a doctorate is the terminal degree needed (that word 'terminal' sounds so final – let's call it your 'likely last but who knows' degree!).

For entry level students, you chose the occupational therapy clinical doctorate versus the master of science degree for a reason. Whatever the reason, you chose a path that will certainly lead to greater knowledge, skill, capacity for clinical reasoning, and, above all else, a degree in a profession for which you can take great pride.

With your new adventure, comes a specific responsibility: to create and complete a doctoral capstone and engage in an immersive doctoral experience. We say adventure because it surely is one. This workbook will take the reader through the many steps of creating the capstone. This includes the formulation of a project, the many stages of development, straight through to writing, and then planning for dissemination. We will also distinguish for you the meaning of the 'capstone project' and 'the doctoral experience'.

We want to emphasize the workbook nature of this book. This workbook is different from other texts in that we provide introductory information for each chapter, and then we provide extensive worksheets and clarify each stage of development of your project. In each chapter you will find at least one worksheet you can utilize for each stage of development of the capstone, including strategies for developing a meaningful experience, disseminating the project in a way that is useful and meaningful for YOU, and planning to sustain the meaningful project you create and put out into the world.

While considering your capstone project, also consider the AOTA Vision 2025 statement:

> As an inclusive profession, occupational therapy maximizes health, well-being, and quality of life for all people, populations, and communities through effective solutions that facilitate participation in everyday living.
>
> (AOTA, 2020)

This vision statement considers all aspects of practice. For a moment, reflect upon this vision statement. Consider the following: Why did you decide to become an occupational therapist and/or pursue a higher level of education? What were your motivations? Was it a single person, or group of people, who inspired you? Was it something in your community that you wanted to enhance, improve or advocate for? Or maybe it was a societal issue that urged you to dig deeper to uncover how you might be of service? The concepts of caring, adaptation, inclusion, diversity, health, well-being, and quality of life, to name but a few, are those that could help you to discover the capstone that is most important and meaningful for you.

DOI: 10.4324/9781003525868-1

As a doctoral student, upon completion of your project and experience, you will:

- Have achieved entry-level competence through a combination of didactic fieldwork and the capstone project and experience.
- Be prepared to evaluate and choose appropriate theories to inform practice.
- Be prepared to articulate and apply therapeutic use of occupations with persons, groups, and populations, for the purpose of facilitating performance and participation in activities, occupations, roles, and situations at your home or school, or in your workplace, community, and other settings, as informed and promoted by the Occupational Therapy Practice Framework (2020).
- Be able to plan and apply evidence-based occupational therapy interventions to address the physical, cognitive, functional cognitive, psychosocial, sensory, and other aspects of performance in a variety of contexts and environments to support engagement in everyday life activities that affect health, well-being, and quality of life, as informed by the Occupational Therapy Practice Framework (2020).
- Be prepared to be a lifelong learner to keep current with evidence-based professional practice.
- Uphold the ethical standards, values, and attitudes of the occupational therapy profession.
- Be prepared to effectively communicate and work interprofessionally with all who provide services and programs for persons, groups, and populations.
- Be prepared to advocate as a professional for access to occupational therapy services offered and for the recipients of those services.
- Be prepared to be an effective consumer of the latest research and knowledge bases that support occupational therapy practice and contribute to the growth and dissemination of research and knowledge.
- Demonstrate in-depth knowledge of delivery models, policies, and systems, related to practice in settings where occupational therapy is currently practiced and settings where it is emerging.
- Demonstrate active involvement in professional development, leadership, and advocacy.
- Demonstrate the ability to synthesize in-depth knowledge in a practice area through the development and completion of a doctoral capstone, in one or more of the following areas: clinical practice skills, research skills, administration, leadership, program and policy development, advocacy, education, and theory development (ACOTE, 2018, Preamble).

The time and effort you take when using this workbook will surely be reflected in your capstone project, and your experience will be that much easier to discover, create, and implement. This workbook will help you both academically and personally, as every project usually comes from a place of caring and the need to educate others about something for which you have great passion. We can't wait to see what you have in store for your profession, your OT program, your community, and society!

REFERENCES

ACOTE (2018). 2018 Accreditation Council for Occupational Therapy Education. https://acoteonline.org/wp-content/uploads/2020/10/2018-ACOTE-Standards.pdf.

American Occupational Therapy Association (AOTA) (2020). Occupational Therapy Practice Framework: Domain and Process. Fourth Edition. *The American Journal of Occupational Therapy*. August, *74*(sup_2), 7412410010p1–7412410010p87. doi: 10.5014/ajot.2020.74S2001.

Why the Occupational Therapy Doctorate (OTD)? And Introduction to Capstone

THE HISTORY OF THE OTD

The occupational therapy doctorate (OTD) can be traced back to 1994, when the first post-professional doctorate program started at Nova Southeastern University, Fort Lauderdale, Florida. Similar to other healthcare professions, and higher education trends, a transition to a clinical doctorate was considered a means to advance the profession. If we look back at the 1980s, we can see a similar attempt to advance the profession.

Reflecting on the progression in occupational therapy (OT) education during the 1980s, there is a noticeable trend: a shift from bachelor's to master's degree programs. Here is a breakdown of the pioneering institutions and the respective leaders who championed the change in entry point from bachelor's to master's level:

First Entry-Level Doctorate Programs

- Creighton University, Omaha, NE
- Washington University, St. Louis, MO
- The University of Toledo, Toledo, OH
- Belmont University, Nashville, TN
- University of the Sciences, Philadelphia, PA

Retrieved from: http://ajot.aota.org/. Terms of use: http://AOTA.org/terms.

Since these original five programs, the number of doctoral programs has increased to over 160 (see Table 1.1). The path from a bachelor's to a master's degree in occupational therapy is comparable to the path from a master's degree to an OTD. Both transitions necessitate a higher level of education and training, and result in increased professional opportunities and responsibilities. The OTD provides a higher level of experience and in-depth understanding and specialization in the field of occupational therapy. The introduction of accredited entry level doctoral programs, again, mirrors broader trends in higher education. As a result, the profession introduced the entry-level doctoral degree as another entry point into the field. By September 1998, we can see the trailblazers championing the addition of the first accredited entry level OTD programs:

- **Southeastern University**

  - Reba Anderson, PhD, OTR/L, FAOTA
  - Suze Dudley, MS, OTR/L, FAOTA

DOI: 10.4324/9781003525868-2

Table 1.1 Number of Programs in the Accreditation Process

Program Status	OTD	OTM	OTA-B	OTA-A	Total
Accreditation	90	167	4	222	483*
Candidate or pre-accreditation	71	11	9	5	96
Applicant	53	22	7	10	92
Total	214	200	20	237	671

Notes: OTM – Occupational therapist master's; OTA-B – Occupational therapy assistant bachelor's; OTA-A – Occupational therapist – associates

*of the total accredited programs, 14 OTM and 9 OTA programs have accreditation-inactive status.

Source: ACOTE (n.d.)

OTD graduates have more career options available to them, in addition to a broader range of skills and knowledge. They can hold positions of leadership in clinical practice, education, research, and administration. They can also contribute to shaping the future of the occupational therapy profession by helping to develop policies, guidelines, and standards. The OTD is a valuable degree for those looking to advance their careers in occupational therapy. It offers a higher level of education and training, which leads to greater expertise and specialization in the field. OTD graduates enter the profession with more career options, such as the aforementioned leadership roles in clinical practice, education, research, and administration. One study found that 64% of OTD students were employed at their capstone experiential site, or a site similar to their experiential site (Kiraly-Alvarez et al., 2022). Knowing this, OTD students should reflect on the population they want to work with after they graduate, and decide how they can plan an experience at the person, group, organization, or community level. (See Learning Activity 1.1).

Use Worksheet 1.1 to reflect on the reasons you selected the OTD, your career goals, and what you would like to accomplish during your OTD capstone. Understanding why you selected this career path can provide insight into the future direction of your capstone.

Worksheet 1.1: Reflection

Goal: Use these reflection questions to select a direction, either a problem or a population, that you would like to pursue for your capstone. (Note: Capstone = project and experience).

1. What personal characteristics and skills do you possess that align with the doctoral program in occupational therapy?

   _____

   _____

   _____

   _____

2. Why did you decide to become an occupational therapist?

_____

_____

_____

_____

3. How do you hope to impact the lives of others through your chosen profession?

_____

_____

_____

_____

4. Why did you choose the doctoral program in occupational therapy over a bachelor's or master's degree?

_____

_____

_____

_____

5. What experiences have confirmed your desire to pursue a career in this field?

_____

_____

_____

_____

6. How do you envision your future in the field of occupational therapy?

_____

_____

_____

_____

7. What are your occupational therapy-related professional objectives?

_____

_____

_____

_____

8. What do you hope to gain from the doctoral program in occupational therapy?

_____

---

9. Have you investigated alternative programs and careers prior to selecting occupational therapy?

---

10. How do you believe the doctoral program in occupational therapy will help you to achieve your long-term objectives and goals?

THE CAPSTONE EXPLORES THE FULL SCOPE OF THE PROFESSION

The OTD capstone allows students to explore the full scope of the profession. The occupational therapy profession has a broad scope that includes a diverse range of populations, settings, and interventions. Occupational therapists work with people of all ages and abilities to help them engage in meaningful and important occupations. Among other things, this includes daily activities such as self-care, work, leisure, and social participation.

Occupational therapists can also work in hospitals, schools, community-based organizations, and private practices. One of the profession's distinguishing features is its emphasis on addressing the individual's holistic needs. This includes not only addressing physical impairments, but also social, emotional, and cognitive factors that can impact an individual's ability to participate in desired occupations. A distinguishing characteristic of the profession to create long-term health and productivity is a focus on health promotion and illness prevention from an individual, community, societal, and global perspective. These areas make for excellent capstone projects, especially in non-traditional settings.

Occupational therapists collaborate with clients, families, and other members of the healthcare team to create interventions specific to the individual's needs and goals. One of the ways that occupational therapy students can add value to the profession is by completing OTD capstone projects that serve non-traditional populations. Non-traditional populations can include individuals who have been traditionally underserved or marginalized, such as individuals experiencing homelessness, LGBT+ youth, individuals with mental health conditions, or individuals with disabilities in low-income countries. By working with non-traditional populations, occupational therapy students can gain a deeper understanding of the unique challenges and barriers that these individuals face and develop

interventions that are better suited to their needs. In addition, students can also gain an understanding of the cultural and social factors that influence occupational performance, which can be critical to provide effective intervention.

The scope of practice for occupational therapists includes providing OT services that are reimbursable by insurance, but also services that are not reimbursable but improve health status. Reimbursable services include assessment, treatment planning, and intervention for conditions such as physical impairments, developmental delays, and chronic health conditions. However, the OTD capstone experience allows students to expand their knowledge and skills beyond this traditional scope of practice. This could include developing interventions that are not typically covered by insurance, such as community-based programs and policy development. These new services from students' capstones can contribute to the development of new models of care that are more readily accessible and equitable for all individuals.

The occupational therapy profession is a dynamic and diverse field that provides students with numerous opportunities to make a positive difference in the lives of individuals and communities.

Students can gain an understanding of the cultural and social factors that influence occupational performance by working with non-traditional populations, which is essential for providing effective care.

IMPORTANCE OF EVIDENCE-INFORMED PRACTICES: APPLY THE SCIENTIFIC METHOD

The scientific method, when applied to an OTD capstone project, provides a structured approach to problem-solving and decision-making. Students can gather and analyze data in a rigorous and systematic manner by following the scientific method, resulting in more valid and reliable conclusions. The scientific method allows for the identification and control of variables, resulting in a more comprehensive understanding of the problem.

The scientific method allows for replication, which adds to the body of evidence in the problem area (National Academies of Sciences, Engineering, and Medicine, 2019). According to Ho et al. (2023), healthcare students who used the scientific method in their OTD capstone projects developed critical thinking skills which were more successful in identifying relevant research and developing effective interventions. Students who used the scientific method to develop their capstone project are also better able to communicate the significance of their findings to stakeholders. Over time, this skill improves societal understanding of the profession.

The ability to replicate a capstone project is an advantage of using the scientific method. Replicability is an important scientific research principle because it allows other researchers to test the validity of a study's findings by conducting their own research using similar methods (National Science Board, 2018). This is especially important in the field of occupational therapy, where intervention effectiveness varies depending on the population studied. Students can apply scientific methods to increase the likelihood that their findings are generalizable to other populations and can be replicated by others.

One of the key benefits of using the scientific method in an OT capstone project is the ability to control extraneous variables and minimize bias. By following a systematic and structured approach, students can ensure that their capstone project is not influenced by personal beliefs or preconceptions. This is particularly important in the field of occupational therapy, where interventions are often tailored to the unique needs of individual clients. By using the scientific method, students can ensure that the interventions they develop are evidence-based and effective.

This workbook will emphasize the significance of employing the scientific method in OTD capstone projects, as this results in more comprehensive and impactful projects and research. The use of scientific methods in OTD capstone projects is valuable, as it provides a structured approach to problem-solving and decision-making. By following the scientific method, students are able to gather and analyze data in a rigorous and systematic manner, leading to more valid and reliable conclusions (Abou-Hanna et al., 2021; Dalim et al., 2022; Ho et al., 2023; Kruse, 2023).

In conclusion, the application of the scientific method to an occupational therapy capstone project is essential for ensuring the validity and reliability of the project and research findings. By finding a problem from current literature, identifying specific variables, minimizing bias, and focusing efforts of the capstone experience and project, students can ensure that they are contributing to the profession of occupational therapy in a meaningful way. Additionally, by following a systematic and structured approach, students can disseminate findings that are replicable and can be used by future students and researchers.

COMPONENTS OF THE CAPSTONE: THE PROJECT AND THE EXPERIENCE

The Accreditation Council for Occupational Therapy Education (ACOTE) is in charge of setting and updating the standards that occupational therapy programs in the U.S. must follow in order to be accredited. As part of these standards, ACOTE gives advice on the kinds of projects that can fulfill the requirements of an OTD capstone. According to ACOTE's standards, the student's capstone must show that they can combine and apply the knowledge, skills, and attitudes they've learned throughout the OTD program to a real-world problem or issue.

The American Occupational Therapy Association (AOTA) gives a broader view of what the OTD capstone is for and what it hopes to achieve. The AOTA website and publications explain the goals of the profession, which include advancing the science and practice of occupational therapy, promoting health and well-being through engagement in meaningful occupations, and advocating for the rights of individuals and groups to participate in desired occupations. These goals can help guide the development of the capstone and make sure it fits with the profession's values and mission.

AOTA also has resources available for students and faculty who are working on OTD capstone projects. These resources include information on evidence-based practice, ethics, and professional development, as well as opportunities to attend conferences and other professional development events. The AOTA Vision 2025 Statement, which explains the association's long-term goals for the profession, can also be used as a guide for creating capstone projects that help advance the science and practice of occupational therapy. The resources provided by both ACOTE (https://acoteonline.org/accreditation-explained/standards/) and AOTA (https://www.aota.org/publications/ot-practice/ot-practice-issues/2022/entry-level-otd-capstone) can help make sure that an OTD capstone project is rigorous, relevant, and in line with the goals and values of the occupational therapy profession.

WHAT ARE THE DIFFERENT PROJECT TYPES?

The term capstone means both the capstone project and the capstone experience.

There are different, specific capstone project types.

You explore more than your project during the experience. This workbook will guide you to plan both.

The doctoral capstone is the final step in completing a doctorate degree in occupational therapy. It is designed to provide students with an in-depth exposure to one or more of the key areas of the profession, including clinical practice skills, research skills, administration, leadership, program and policy development, advocacy, education, and theory development. By completing a capstone project, students have the opportunity to demonstrate their mastery of the knowledge and skills required to be successful occupational therapists.

Worksheet 1.2 explores each project type. As you read the literature consider which project type would best meet your personal and professional goals from Worksheet 1.1.

Worksheet 1.2: Planning a Project Type

There are eight project types. Use this worksheet to think about considerations for a few (or all) of the project types. Use your current level of knowledge, and understanding of the literature, to explore the project types.

Project Type 1: Clinical Practice Skills

1. For your chosen population, what evidence-based interventions have been shown to be effective in meeting the needs of the population or problem you chose?

   _____

   _____

   _____

   _____

2. For your chosen population, what specific clinical practice skill needs further evidence or development?

   _____

   _____

   _____

   _____

3. For your chosen population, what are the options to advance the understanding or application of a clinical practice skill?

   _____

   _____

   _____

   _____

4. How will you find evidence from the literature that supports the direction your program will take?

   _____

   _____

   _____

   _____

5. Is this achievable in 14 weeks?

_____

Project Type 2: Research Skills

1. For your chosen population or problem, what research questions could be asked to learn more about the population or problem?

_____

_____

_____

_____

2. For your chosen population or problem, what is known about the current recommendations for future research?

_____

_____

_____

_____

3. For your chosen population or problem, how will you plan and carry out a research study to find the answers to your questions?

_____

_____

_____

_____

4. For your chosen population or problem, how will you find evidence from the literature that supports this direction for your project type?

_____

_____

_____

_____

5. Is this achievable in 14 weeks?

_____

Project Type 3: Administration

1. For your chosen population, what administrative problems do providers have to deal with when caring for this group or solving this problem?

_____

_____

_____

_____

2. For your chosen population, what is known about the current administrative challenges?

_____

_____

_____

_____

3. For your chosen population, how can you come up with and use plans, or build on what is currently known to deal with these problems?

_____

_____

_____

_____

4. For your chosen population, how will you find evidence from the literature that supports this direction for your project type?

_____

_____

_____

_____

5. Is this achievable in 14 weeks?

_____

Project Type 4: Leadership

1. For your chosen population, how can you show leadership by working to improve the lives of this group or solving this problem?

_____

_____

_____

_____

2. For your chosen population, what is known about the current leadership challenges?

_____

_____

_____

_____

3. For your chosen population, how can you get other people involved and work together to reach this goal?

_____

_____

_____

_____

4. How will you find evidence from the literature that supports this direction for your project type?

_____

_____

_____

_____

5. Is this achievable in 14 weeks?

_____

Project Type 5: Program and Policy Development

1. What programs and policies are there to help this group of people or this problem?

_____

_____

_____

_____

2. For your chosen population, what is known about the current challenges related to program and policy development?

_____

_____

_____

_____

3. For your chosen population, how can you come up with and use new programs or policies to make things better?

_____

_____

_____

_____

4. For your chosen population, how will you find evidence from the literature that supports this direction for your project type?

_____

_____

_____

_____

5. Is this achievable in 14 weeks?

_____

Project Type 6: Advocacy

1. What organizations and advocacy efforts are available to help this group of people or this problem?

_____

_____

_____

_____

2. For your chosen population, what is known about the current challenges related to advocacy? What are specific advocacy goals for the population or problem?

_____

_____

_____

_____

3. For your chosen population, what can you do to support advocacy efforts for this group's needs and rights or to solve this problem?

_____

_____

_____

_____

4. How will you find evidence from the literature that supports this direction for your project type?

_____

_____

_____

_____

5. Is this achievable in 14 weeks?

_____

Project Type 7: Education

1. For your chosen population, what is known about existing educational offerings to help this group of people or this problem?

_____

_____

_____

_____

2. For your chosen population, what is known about the current challenges related to education, or gaps in educational offerings?

_____

_____

_____

_____

3. For your chosen population, how can you come up with and deliver educational offerings?

_____

_____

_____

_____

4. For your chosen population, how will you find evidence from the literature that supports this direction for your project type?

_____

_____

_____

_____

5. Is this achievable in 14 weeks?

_____

Project Type 8: Theory Development

1. For your chosen population, what theories or models can help you better understand this group of people or this problem?

_____

_____

_____

_____

2. For your chosen population, what is known about the current challenges related to theory and theory development?

_____

_____

_____

_____

3. For your chosen population, how can you develop or refine theories that can inform practice, research, or advocacy efforts?

_____

_____

_____

_____

4. For your chosen population, how will you find evidence from the literature that supports this direction for your project type?

_____

_____

_____

_____

5. Is this achievable in 14 weeks?

_____

THE EXPERIENCE

As part of their OTD program, students will spend 14 weeks in an individual supervised and mentored practice setting. Even though the project doesn't have to be done at the mentored practice setting, the experience must show how the knowledge learned throughout the capstone development process was put together and used. For instance, consider the following scenario: A student is running a program in a community setting, such as for a weekly arthritis support group. The primary objectives for this project would occur at the arthritis support group, but the experience would be at a different organization that serves the same population such as the Arthritis Foundation or a private rheumatology practice. This approach broadens the student's exposure to and understanding of their area of focus by providing the opportunity to work with the populations at two different service levels.

Finding and securing a mentored practice setting should be fun because it gives you a chance to explore areas of interest and work with different kinds of people or projects. Students should choose sites that will give them the most experience with the group or type of project they are interested in. This could mean doing research on possible places to work, talking to mentors or peers, or searching the internet for locations that address the designated problem or population of interest. Students who are in programs where their Doctoral Capstone Coordinator (DCC) finds a site for them should supply the DCC with a sufficient number of sites to explore. These sites should be those at which the student would definitely want to have their capstone experience, so proper vetting by the student is required prior to submitting to the DCC.

Once a mentored practice setting has been found, students will work closely with their doctoral coordinator and mentor to come up with specific goals and a plan for supervision. This could mean figuring out where the student needs more help or needs to improve their skills, as well as listing the activities and experiences that will ensure the student reaches their goals. Throughout the experience, the mentor will help guide and support the student by giving feedback, advice, and the opportunity to work towards the desired goals.

During the mentored practice experience, students will be able to use the knowledge and skills they have learned throughout the program. This could mean the objectives planned for the experience can come from other project-type categories. For example, during the experience, you could work with patients, do research, make programs or policies, or get involved in activities like advocacy or education. Despite these not being the primary project type, by taking part in these activities, students will be able to show that they can combine and apply knowledge in a meaningful way while gaining valuable experience in a real-world setting.

In short, the capstone experience or mentored practice experience gives students a chance to work with the population or project type of their choice while setting specific goals and making plans for supervision. Students will be able to use what they have learned in the real world, with the help of their mentor, to take part in activities that show how they can combine and apply what they have learned.

Use Worksheet 1.3 to begin thinking about how you will pick your mentored practice setting.

Worksheet 1.3: Considerations for the Capstone Experience or Mentored Practice Setting

The capstone experience takes place in a mentored setting. It is 14 weeks, full time, with flexibility to plan off-mentored practice setting activities.

Goal: Use these reflection questions to consider direction for the experiential component of the capstone. Consider sites that support the problem or population identified. Reflect on where you can gain an in-depth exposure at a person, organization, population, or community level.

1. What is my area of interest, and how can I find a mentored practice setting that would provide me with in-depth exposure to my area of interest?

   _____

   _____

   _____

   _____

2. What kinds of people or projects do I want to learn more about during my capstone experience?

   _____

_____
_____
_____

3. What are the specific goals and learning outcomes I want to accomplish during my capstone experience?

_____
_____
_____
_____

4. What resources and chances will I have to grow as a professional at each possible setting for my capstone experience?

_____
_____
_____
_____

5. How does the identified mentored practice setting fit with my personal and professional goals?

_____
_____
_____
_____

6. Where is each possible mentored practice setting and how easy is it to get to? How does this fit with my personal and logistical needs?

_____
_____
_____
_____

7. What is the timeline and availability for each possible mentored practice setting, and how does this fit with my program requirements and personal schedule?

_____
_____
_____
_____

8. What questions do I have for potential mentors or current students at each mentored practice setting, and how can I get the best information to make an informed decision?

_____

_____

_____

_____

Learning Activity 1.1: Planning the Project and Experience for Persons, Groups, and Populations

- **Introduction**

  o Instructions: Reflect on the population you wish to work with during your capstone. Consider how you can plan impactful experiences at different levels – personal, group, organizational, and community.

- **Identifying the Population**

- **Describe the Population:**

  o Who are they? (e.g., age group, specific needs, interests)
  o What are their primary challenges or needs?

- **Why this Population?**

  o Explain your interest in working with this population.
  o How does this align with your career goals?

- **Option 1: Person/Individual Level Engagement (if you chose your capstone to focus at the personal/individual level):**

  o Direct interaction:

    - What kind of direct, one-on-one experiences could you provide?
    - Where would you be able to provide these services or experiences outside of traditional practice, since the capstone experience cannot be a third level II?
    - How would these experiences benefit the individual?

  o Personal development goals:

    - What skills or knowledge do you hope to gain from providing one-on-one interactions?
    - How will you measure the success of these individual interactions?
    - What challenges do you anticipate at the individual level?

- **Option 2: Group-Level Engagement**

  o Group-level activities:

    - What are potential group activities or programs you could develop?
    - How will these activities address the group's needs?
    - Where would you be able to provide these services at a group level?

- o Personal development goals:
  - What skills or knowledge do you hope to gain from completing your capstone to a group?
  - How will you measure the success of these group interactions?
  - How will you facilitate positive group dynamics?
  - What challenges do you anticipate in group settings?

- **Option 3: Organizational-Level Engagement**

  - o Organizational-level activities:
    - Identify potential organizations for collaboration.
    - How will these collaborations enhance your work with the population?
    - What impact do you hope to have at the organizational level?
    - How will you evaluate the effectiveness of your organizational engagement?

  - o Personal development goals:
    - What skills or knowledge do you hope to gain from completing your capstone working at the organizational level?
    - How will you measure the success of your capstone on the organization?
    - What challenges do you anticipate at the organizational level?

- **Option 4: Community-Level Engagement**

  - o Community initiatives:
    - Identify community-level initiatives or programs.
    - How do these initiatives meet community needs?
  - o Personal development goals:
    - What skills or knowledge do you hope to gain from completing your capstone working at the community level?
    - How will you measure the success of your capstone on the community?
    - What challenges do you anticipate at the community level?

- **Reflection and Action Plan**

  - o Summarize your key reflections from each section.
  - o Create an action plan with steps to implement your ideas at each level.
  - o How would engaging in more than one level of involvement enrich your capstone experience?

REFERENCES

Abou-Hanna, J. J., Owens, S. T., Kinnucan, J. A., Mian, S. I., & Kolars, J. C. (2021). Resuscitating the Socratic Method: Student and Faculty Perspectives on Posing Probing Questions during Clinical Teaching. *Academic Medicine, 96*(1), 113–117.

ACOTE (n.d.). Schools. Retrieved from: https://acoteonline.org/all-schools.

American Occupational Therapy Association (2016). OTD Impact Study. Retrieved from: https://www.aota.org/Education-Careers/Accreditation/OTD-Impact-Study.aspx.

American Occupational Therapy Association (2020a). Occupational Therapy Doctoral Degree. Retrieved from: https://www.aota.org/Education-Careers/Students-Residents/Doctoral-Degree.

American Occupational Therapy Association (2020b). OTD Competencies. Retrieved from: https://www.aota.org/Education-Careers/Accreditation/.

American Occupational Therapy Association (2021a). Occupational Therapy Practice Framework: Domain and Process (4th ed.). *American Journal of Occupational Therapy*, 75(sup_1), S1–S48. https://doi.org/10.5014/ajot.2021.75S1.

American Occupational Therapy Association (2021b). Occupational Therapy in Non-Traditional Settings. Retrieved from: https://www.aota.org/-/media/Corporate/Files/AboutOT/Professionals/Non-Traditional-Settings.pdf.

Andersen, L. T., & Reed, K. L. (2017). *The History of Occupational Therapy: The First Century*. SLACK Incorporated.

Dalim, S. F., Ishak, A. S., & Hamzah, L. M. (2022). Promoting Students' Critical Thinking Through Socratic Method: The Views and Challenges. *Asian Journal of University Education*, 18(4), 1034–1047.

Ho, Y. R., Chen, B. Y., & Li, C. M. (2023). Thinking More Wisely: Using the Socratic Method to Develop Critical Thinking Skills amongst Healthcare Students. *BMC Medical Education*, 23(1), 173.

Kemp, E., Domina, A., Delbert, T., Rivera, A., & Navarro-Walker, L. (2020). Development, Implementation and Evaluation of Entry-Level Occupational Therapy Doctoral Capstones: A National Survey. *Journal of Occupational Therapy Education*, 4(4). https://doi.org/10.26681/jote.2020.040411.

Kemp, E. L., Domina, A., Stephenson, S., & Start, A. (2022). Perceived Value & Usefulness of the Entry-Level Occupational Therapy Doctoral Capstone. *Journal of Occupational Therapy Education*, 6(3). https://doi.org/10.26681/jote.2022.060311.

Kiraly-Alvarez, A. F., Clegg, A., Lucas Molitor, W., & Friberg, D. (2022). An Exploration of the Occupational Therapy Doctoral Capstone: Perspectives from Capstone Coordinators, Graduates, and Site Mentors. *Journal of Occupational Therapy Education*, 6(1). https://doi.org/10.26681/jote.2022.060114.

Krueger, R. B., Sweetman, M. M., Martin, M., & Cappaert, T. A. (2020). Occupational Therapists' Implementation of Evidence-Based Practice: A Cross Sectional Survey. *Occupational Therapy in Health Care*, 34(3), 253–276.

Kruse, S. (2023, February 23). The Socratic Method: Fostering Critical Thinking. The Institute for Learning and Teaching. Retrieved from: https://tilt.colostate.edu/the-socratic-method/.

National Academies of Sciences, Engineering, and Medicine (2019). Replicability. In *Reproducibility and Replicability in Science* (pp. 77–95). The National Academies Press.

National Science Board (2018). Science and Engineering Indicators 2018 (NSB-2018–1). Retrieved from: https://www.nsf.gov/statistics/2018/nsb20181/report.

Needs Assessment

Lisa Bagby

In this chapter, we will break down what a needs assessment is, when a needs assessment is necessary, what a needs assessment means for doctoral capstone project planning, and how a needs assessment helps us make decisions. Let's start by defining each word as it relates to the process of needs assessment. Merriam-Webster (2023) defines 'need' and 'assessment' as the following:

Need, noun

2a: a lack of something requisite, desirable, or useful
2b: a physiological or psychological requirement for the well-being of an organism
3: a condition requiring supply or relief

Assessment, noun

1: the action or an instance of making a judgment about something: the act of assessing something

WHAT IS A NEEDS ASSESSMENT?

When we combine the above definitions, a needs assessment is the act of assessing, or making a judgment, about whether a person, condition, or circumstance is lacking, or could benefit from something desirable, useful, or relieving. Simply, a needs assessment is the act of *assessing* the *needs* of a situation, organization, or population in order to identify the gap between their current resources and their desired goals or outcomes.

Throughout your life, you have likely completed more needs assessments than you could reasonably count. As humans, we assess our own needs, needs of others, needs related to our roles, and needs of many other situations and circumstances daily without significant thought or difficulty. For example, I may ask my friends if they need me to pick anything up for a birthday party they are hosting, and they request I bring candles for the cake. On this small scale, I have identified where a gap existed (lack of candles) and a desired outcome (having candles on the cake for a celebration). Similarly, as OTs we complete needs assessments multiple times per day ranging from informal observations to thorough evaluations and in-depth analyses in order to identify what our clients' desired outcomes or goals may be and where the gaps or challenges are which may impact their ability to reach those goals. The needs assessment process is happening around us all the time.

Needs assessments vary from simple to complex and from one-time occurrences to ongoing assessment cycles. The type of needs assessment completed is dependent upon a multitude of factors, such as your overarching purpose or goal, the environment and/or context, the stakeholders involved, and timeline. Bradshaw (1972) developed the 'Taxonomy of Social Need,' in which he identifies and qualifies four types of needs: 1) normative need, 2) felt need, 3) expressed need, and 4) comparative

DOI: 10.4324/9781003525868-3

need. *Normative need* is identified by an expert or authority and is the comparison between a desired standard and what actually exists, frequently driven by data or research. For instance, Azevedo et al. (2022) identified after-school programming as an effective strategy for reducing educational inequality, which was exacerbated by the COVID-19 pandemic. *Felt need* is a need which the population being assessed *feels* they need. An example of this would be parents feeling like their children need greater after-school resources since falling behind in the wake of the pandemic. *Expressed need* is the felt need in action. This looks like the same group of parents from the example above acting and going to a school board meeting to advocate for increased after-school offerings. Finally, *comparative need* is assessed by comparing groups with similar characteristics in relationship to a service. Continuing with the after-school program example, if a community has five elementary schools and three of the schools have robust after-school programming while two do not, despite the same student demographics and needs, the comparative need indicates increased after-school programming offerings for the two schools where programming is less robust.

While we will not go into further depth with Bradshaw's (1972) taxonomy, it is important to start conceptualizing various systematic approaches for completing needs assessments in your future work. Since the primary objective of this chapter is to provide you with context and structure to ensure you meet the standards for doctoral

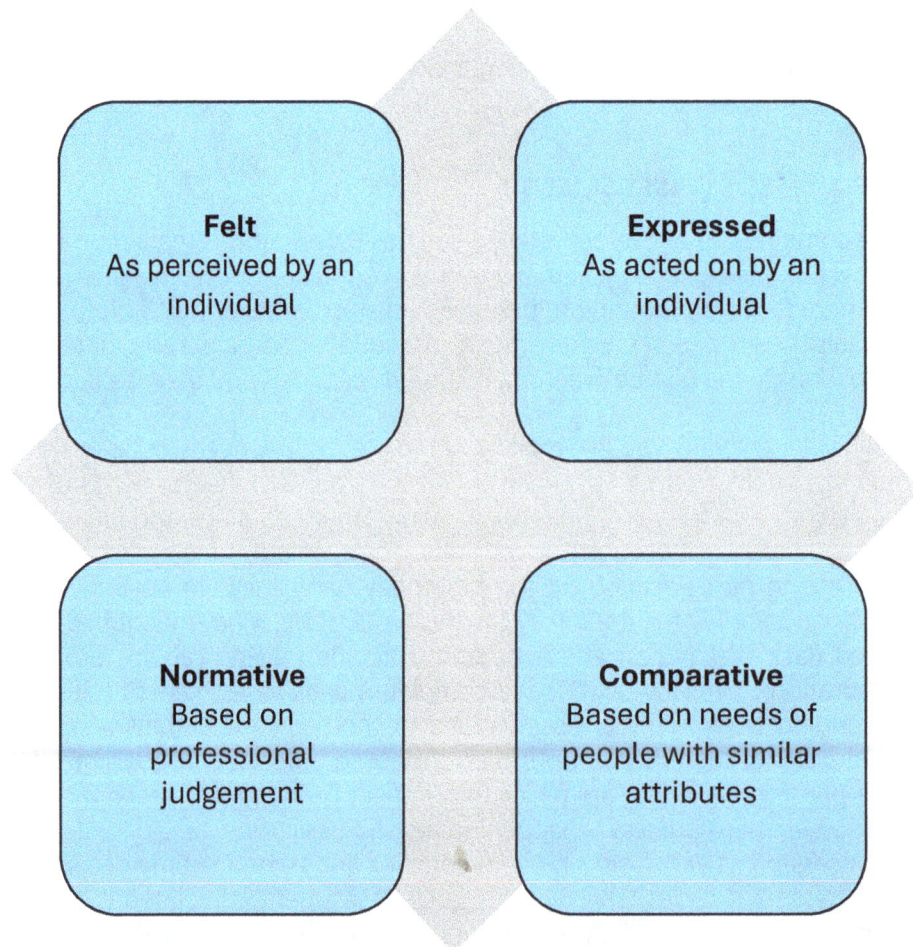

Felt
As perceived by an individual

Expressed
As acted on by an individual

Normative
Based on professional judgement

Comparative
Based on needs of people with similar attributes

Figure 2.1 Social Need Taxonomy

Source: Bradshaw's (1972) Social Need Taxonomy from Tweed (2016)

capstone project planning (ACOTE, 2018), we will predominantly focus on normative and comparative needs, which closely align with the capstone planning needs assessment process.

NEEDS ASSESSMENT AND DOCTORAL CAPSTONE PROJECT PLANNING

There are a few questions related to the needs assessment standard that you may be asking yourself or your Doctoral Capstone Coordinator (DCC), as you embark on your capstone planning journey, such as:

- What is the purpose of a needs assessment in doctoral capstone project planning?
- If the capstone is focused on the students' desired learning, why is a needs assessment relevant or necessary?
- What is the difference between completing a needs assessment in the planning phase of capstone versus after the capstone has started?

Understanding the rationale and purpose for completing a needs assessment for doctoral capstone planning is one of the key elements for ensuring your capstone experience and project are as relevant and successful as possible. The primary rationale for completing a needs assessment during the capstone project planning process is to affirm if the knowledge you seek to gain through the capstone is relevant. If we think about what the capstone is in OT education, we know it is an opportunity for students to do a deep dive into an area of their interest, synthesizing didactic and clinical experiences, in new or novel ways. With this in mind, the purpose of completing a needs assessment during the planning process is to ensure your focus area and the population you choose to explore is necessary, relevant, and timely to advance knowledge within the profession.

Consider this example: You decide to focus your capstone on clinical practice skills, with a plan to work with adults in hand therapy. You do a search to find the number of clinicians in the geographic area where you want to complete your capstone experience. In your research, you find there are 1,000 clinicians in the area and 500 of those clinicians are hand therapists. With this information, do you think there is a need for you to study or explore clinical practice skills related to hand therapy in this geographic area? Probably not. Conversely, consider you find out there are only five hand therapists out of 10,000 clinicians in the geographic area. Is there a need to explore clinical practice skills related to hand therapy with this new information? The answer to this question is . . . *maybe*. What additional information do you think would be necessary to know, definitively, whether a hand therapy-focused capstone experience would be necessary, relevant, and timely for the population within your chosen geographic area? Would you like to seek information about common industries in the area? Or the number of people who have hand injuries each year? If there are only five hand therapists, are all of them CHTs? What are the therapists' practice experiences and expertise?

While the capstone experience and project are based upon students' desired learning, part of doctoral education and professionalism requires development of skills to discern when and if your work and actions benefit the population(s) you serve and the profession at large. The needs assessment step in capstone planning is a built-in opportunity to learn and practice these vital skills to prepare you for entering the OT workforce. Your time in the clinic will, predominantly, be spent in providing patient care, completing documentation, and ensuring you meet productivity expectations. When taking on new projects or leadership roles in your career, understanding the importance of evaluating whether a project is warranted and feasible before starting can save you time and money in the long run.

As occupational therapists, we assess our clients' needs and the needs of other people, populations, groups, situations, and organizations. So how do we know what type of needs assessment we should do to plan the capstone project versus the type of needs assessment we can do after starting the capstone experience? The simple answer is we have to consider the purpose and/or desired outcome. However, it is a bit more complex than this. An initial needs assessment is required while planning the project to determine if the project is worth pursuing. Once the capstone experience begins, another needs assessment can be carried out to shape and/or modify the project or experiential objectives. The required initial needs assessment focuses on, and informs, whether we should pursue a project, and subsequent needs assessments focus on, and inform, how the project could be shaped and implemented. Since the purpose of each is very distinct, we should revisit the types of needs identified in Bradshaw's (1972) taxonomy: normative, expressed, felt, and comparative needs (see Figure 2.1).

Unless you are intimately associated with your chosen capstone site prior to the start of your capstone planning, the likelihood of you having access to and understanding of the expressed or felt needs of the organization or population is unlikely. Therefore, the needs assessment completed during the capstone planning process will likely remain in the realm of normative and comparative needs, which is information you can gather, or find, through literature and resource review. In a way, the project needs assessment completed during capstone planning is a preliminary needs assessment to inform whether a full needs assessment is necessary. Ideally, you have a site already in mind; performing a needs assessment at the site can have an enormous positive impact on your project and experience. The results can also help you determine how best to utilize the time in your experience to help the organization where you are placed.

Needs Assessment Questions You Should Be Asking as You Embark on Your Doctoral Capstone Planning

1. What is (are) your focus area(s) for your capstone?
   a. Is it directly or indirectly related to OT?
   b. If not directly related, how will you relate the focus of your doctoral capstone to OT?
2. What is the population you want to work with?
   a. How many people in your chosen geographic area are part of your targeted population? i.e., (using hand therapy example above) how many people have hand injuries requiring skilled therapy?
   b. How does your focus area address the needs of your target population?
   c. What other populations have similar experiences?
   d. Is there a comparative need between this population and another group with similar characteristics?
3. If you have more than one area of focus and/or more than one targeted population, how are you tying your focus together?
   a. Do you have an overarching theme for your learning?
      (If not, this is an important aspect of ensuring all your work is moving toward the same goal).
   b. Does one area of focus inform the other? i.e., do you need to complete one aspect in order to complete the next?
   c. If you must complete one aspect first, what is the order you would need to follow? What is your rationale for this?
   d. Are you able to work on all focus areas simultaneously?

4. What are you specifically wanting to learn in relation to your focus area(s) and population(s)?
   a. Is my focus too broad? Why/why not?
      i. If yes, how can I make it more specific/attainable?
   b. Is my focus too narrow? Why/why not?
      i. If yes, how can I make it more encompassing of the needs of the population I'm working with?
5. Are there occupational therapists working in this space?
   a. If yes, how many OTs are working in this sector?
   b. If yes, how many OTs are doing this work in the geographic area I am planning to work in?
   c. If not, who is a subject matter expert in this space who could help inform your capstone?
6. What other professionals are present in this space?
   a. Are they working with or addressing the particular area of need you are focused on with this population?
   b. If yes, what are they doing and how are they addressing the need?
   c. How is what you would do, from an OT perspective, different from what is being done in this space or sector?
7. What do you want to learn/what skills do you want to develop (broadly) by the end of your capstone experience and project?
   a. Is there literature to help support how you approach learning?
8. Is there literature to support your area(s) of focus?
   a. If not, is there adjacent, or partially related, literature to your area(s) of focus that you could generalize to your focus area?
      i. If there is partially related literature, how will you demonstrate the connection to your area(s) of focus?
      ii. If you are unable to find supporting literature, is this the best focus area to pursue?
   b. Has your review of the literature indicated a normative need to study this focus area?
   c. Has your review of the literature indicated a normative need for working with your selected population in this focus area?
   d. Is there literature outlining the experiences of a comparable population to demonstrate a comparative need?
   e. Is there literature to support comparable areas of focus if literature is not available for the specific sector you are pursuing? (e.g., OT and accessibility in various sectors [transportation, interior design, public spaces such as museums, theaters, etc.]).
   f. Is there literature/data related to your desired outcome?
      i. If yes, how will you incorporate what you learn from the literature into your capstone plan?
      ii. If not, is there literature/data adjacent to your desired outcome that could be applied to your capstone?
9. As you've gathered information, what is the overarching need for you to explore your focus area(s) for your doctoral capstone experience and project?
10. Did you find enough evidence that you should move forward with this doctoral capstone idea?
11. What is your vision for how studying this will create a lasting impact on the population you want to work with and the OT profession?

NEEDS ASSESSMENTS AND DECISION-MAKING

Needs assessments, especially when completed in a systematic way, provide us with an incredible amount of information. Once we have gathered the relevant information regarding the normative, felt, expressed, and comparative needs of our project, we have a greater and more informed perspective to make decisions about the direction we want to take, or the direction we *should* take. Needs assessments help to inform how we structure our projects; assisting in making a road map for where we want to go next. For capstone planning, the preliminary needs assessment helps you to decide whether or not you should study and expand your knowledge in a particular area or focus and is a great starting point for setting you up for an informed, relevant, and impactful doctoral capstone experience.

REFERENCES

Accreditation Council for Occupational Therapy Education (ACOTE) (2018). Standards and Interpretive Guide (effective July 31, 2020). *The American Journal of Occupational Therapy, 72*(sup_2), 7212410005p1–7212410005p83. https://doi.org/10.5014/ajot.2018.72S217.

Azevedo, J. P., Gutierrez, M., de Hoyos, R., & Saavedra, J. (2022). Chapter 16: The Unequal Impacts of COVID-19 on Student Learning. In F. M. Reimers (ed.), *Primary and Secondary Education During Covid-19*. Springer.

Bradshaw, J. (1972). Taxonomy of Social Need. In G. McLachlan (ed.), *Problems and Progress in Medical Care: Essays On Current Research*. Oxford University Press, pp. 71–82.

Merriam-Webster (2023). 'Need' and 'Assessment'. Retrieved from: https://www.merriam-webster.com/dictionary/need and https://www.merriam-webster.com/dictionary/assessment.

Tweed, E. (2016). *Taking Away the Chaos – The Health Needs of People Who Inject Drugs in Public Places in Glasgow City Center*. Glasgow Centre for Population Health. Retrieved from: https://www.stor.scot.nhs.uk/handle/11289/579845.

Finding and Developing a Problem Worth Pursuing and Relevant to the Profession of Occupational Therapy

In the age of fake news, it is more important than ever to be accurate and factual. When students are given the responsibility of creating and defending a project, project type, and developing a worthwhile experience, they must dedicate time to developing foundational knowledge about the area of interest. A student who is knowledgeable about a topic area will be able to develop arguments for and against a topic area. To get to this level of understanding, it is essential to first research and explore a variety of reputable sources to find detailed, accurate data.

When you take the time to search for reliable information on your topic, not only will you provide the necessary details for your future reader, but you will also learn more about the subject than if you had just relied on your own experience or opinions. By using facts and statistics from reputable sources instead of what just 'seems' correct or their own personal opinions, students will be able to support their arguments against other points of view.

USE ACCURATE INFORMATION FROM REPUTABLE SOURCES

Learning about a topic from a variety of perspectives, both within and outside of OT, is helpful to develop an understanding of a topic area and learn what subject matter experts are currently researching. However, with some careful planning and consideration, the time spent researching a phenomenon can be completed with more efficiency. Suggestions for minimum number and types of primary source evidence to justify the pursuit of a problem include:

Table 3.1 Minimum Number and Types of Primary Source Evidence

Literature type	Proposed minimum number of articles per category to develop an understanding of the area of interest	What is your minimum goal?
Quantitative articles – peer review	3	
Qualitative articles – peer review	3	
Systematic review or meta-analysis	1	
International study	1	
Book – edited academic book or book by someone with the lived experience	1	

(Continued)

Table 3.1 (Continued)

Literature type	Proposed minimum number of articles per category to develop an understanding of the area of interest	What is your minimum goal?
Website material from professional associations	Rarely, use to develop an understanding, but not to support the problem or purpose	

Quantitative Studies

Quantitative studies collect objective data and *analyze for relationships between variables*. By reading at least three quantitative studies, a student can learn the variables that are currently being studied. Alignment with other subject matter experts regarding variables worth studying teaches the student a direction for their project.

Qualitative Studies

Qualitative studies collect information that cannot easily be organized into numerical data. Qualitative studies explore phenomena to develop a deeper understanding. Reading at least three qualitative studies allows the student to develop a deeper understanding of the phenomena as well as learn about the types of exploration currently being conducted. Aligning the capstone with other authors and subject matter experts regarding how a problem could be approached demonstrates critical thinking and increases the likelihood the capstone will be impactful.

Systematic Review of the Literature

A systematic review of the literature is a thorough and methodical way to look at and combine the research studies that have already been done on a certain topic. It means searching for, choosing, and judging relevant studies in a planned way to answer a specific research question. The process follows a set of rules that have already been set up. This makes sure that everything is clear and that bias is kept to a minimum. Through a systematic review, researchers try to give an unbiased summary of the available evidence, find knowledge gaps, and come to useful conclusions about the topic being studied. In the end, the goal of a systematic review is to give a solid and reliable overview of the literature on a certain topic. Finding a systematic review on a topic of interest is a strong way to start a literature review, since you can look up the articles identified in the review to learn more about the current problem.

International Study

Students and faculty can contemplate the number of international studies to use in the development of the capstone project. There are many differences in the context of healthcare delivery that must be taken into consideration when reading international studies. However, there is value in learning about challenges other countries are addressing and comparing the challenges to those in the United States. There are populations, including in mental health, prison, wellness, and education systems, where other countries have better health outcomes than the United States. When researching how to find and disseminate best practices, those practices may already have evidence in other countries.

Books

A book provides an in-depth description and explanation of populations and experiences. Reading a book about a population or societal problem can deepen the student's understanding of the context and lived experiences of an author. Care must be taken when reading a book, to remember that the book is an opinion of a person who has experienced or studied the phenomena. Current research must be read to ensure an accurate approach to address the population or problem.

The source examples provided in Table 3.1 are a minimum list of sources for all students to use when researching topics before drafting a capstone. The next sections describe strategies for collecting and organizing sources so that they can be used to support the project.

WHAT HAPPENS IF I CAN'T FIND LITERATURE ON MY TOPIC OF INTEREST?

In today's world of information overload, there may be a few reasons that you were not able to find the necessary number of primary sources for your project.

One reason you may not be finding current literature is that the terminology had changed, and the search terms being used are outdated. A good example is the use of the term 'sensory integration' as a disorder. If the term sensory integration disorder is Googled, you will find websites describing and defining sensory integration, but it is no longer a disorder. The term may even be in your textbooks as a disorder. However, this term is not found in the *Diagnostic and Statistical Manual of Mental Disorders* (*DSM*) and neither is sensory processing disorder. What changed? In 2012 a policy statement was published outlining why the American Academy of Pediatrics (AAP) should avoid using sensory integrative disorder, and sensory processing disorder, as the primary diagnosis (Zimmer et al., 2012). There may be professionals that disagree with this decision, and the decision may be changed as further evidence is collected. However, the most current literature must be utilized in support of capstone projects rather than hanging one's hat on the opinions of a small number of professionals.

Another reason you are not finding literature on your topic of interest may be that you have only checked for the sources using specific key words. Explore literature published by many disciplines. Occupational therapy was founded by professionals in many different fields. Literature from other disciplines can be scaffolded to link your topic to current literature. Even though your specific area of interest may not be studied directly, it may still be possible to develop a linkage. For example, you may want to develop a capstone project and experience around services for the refugee population. There may not be literature that directly supports occupational therapy services to this population. However, the support can be built by finding current research literature that outlines the known occupational performance issues of refugees. The current literature may support poor cognitive, psychosocial, and mental health outcomes for refugee populations. Next, find the current evidence from the literature that describes successful outcomes of services provided to other populations to improve cognitive, psychosocial, and mental health for these populations. Then make the summary statement that since occupational therapy services demonstrate evidence to support evaluation and intervention for a similar population, further exploration to provide these services to the new population is warranted.

Therefore, don't come to the conclusion quickly that there is no literature on your topic of interest. Rather, try to broaden your thinking concerning what you might need and utilize. You should map the potential areas that are connected to your topic and organize them, through skimming as well as taking notes on what is more relevant and related. Afterward, bring the selected literature together in a manner that backs your selected research topic.

If you cannot find literature on your topic, you can pose these questions to yourself: What else is pertinent? Could the topic be related to a broader problem?

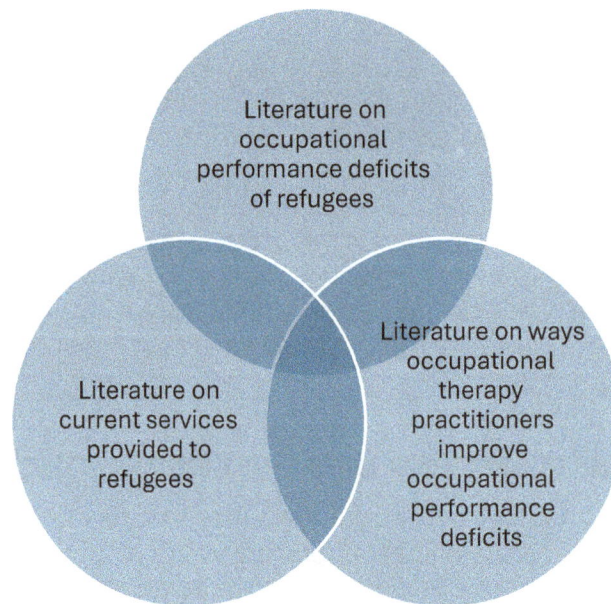

Figure 3.1 Mental Map to Identify Literature to Support an Area of Interest

Note: The center is the role of the OT to improve known occupational performance deficits of refugees, and how OTs can be integrated into the current service delivery model.

Does the topic contribute to something larger in some way? A resulting strategy would be to widen the search boundaries to incorporate framing and related terms.

However, in the case that you decide to pursue your topic despite the lack of literature on it, you must think about who will be interested in it, seeing as it is a new topic. Other academics and professionals will judge the value of your work, be it through peer review or defense. Your time and efforts will be best spent finding a way to link your interests to problems that other academics and professionals are working on.

ENSURE THE PROJECT ENRICHES THE PROFESSION OF OCCUPATIONAL THERAPY

Occupational therapists make a unique contribution to improving the health of individuals, organizations, and populations. The unique perspective is participation in meaningful occupations and varied activities improving health.

As an OTD student, you will have been learning about theories, models, and practices in occupational therapy that have been proven to work. The capstone project is a summary of everything you have learned and a chance to show how well you can use this in the real world.

By explicitly linking occupational therapy to your capstone project, you can improve health through participation in occupation, ensure a chance to show off your knowledge and critical thinking skills, and also help the occupational therapy field move forward.

Being in an OTD program does not automatically link your project to the profession. An OTD project advances the profession in a small, yet meaningful way. It must also be remembered that some problems exist that are not best resolved by occupational therapy.

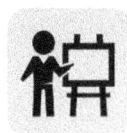

Worksheet Example 3.1: Selecting a Relevant Problem from the Literature

This is an example of finding an area of interest, and finding a need for OTs within that area.

Area of interest: Individuals with Autism Spectrum Disorder (ASD)

A Problem that Can be Found in the Literature Is

The problem is the misdiagnosis of individuals with Autism Spectrum Disorder (ASD), leading to incorrect identification and inadequate support (Fusar-Poli et al., 2022; Takara et al., 2015).

Although this is a problem, occupational therapists do not diagnose individuals with autism. The next step would be, using the Literature Review Grid in Chapter 4 of this workbook, to see if we can begin to link this problem to the profession of OT.

Article Citation in APA

1. Fusar-Poli, L., Brondino, N., Politi, P., & Aguglia, E. (2022). Missed Diagnoses and Misdiagnoses of Adults with Autism Spectrum Disorder. *European Archives of Psychiatry and Clinical Neuroscience, 272*(2), 187–198.
2. Takara, K., Kondo, T., & Kuba, T. (2015). How and Why Is Autism Spectrum Disorder Misdiagnosed in Adult Patients?: From Diagnostic Problem to Management for Adjustment. *Mental Health in Family Medicine, 11*(2), 73–88.

What Questions Did the Author Answer?

We conducted a search of databases (PubMed, PsycINFO, and ERIC) for relevant articles published from January 2000 to May 2015 and summarized unrecognized or misdiagnosed cases as well as major psychiatric comorbidities among adults with ASD from previous reports. Evaluate the psychiatric history of a group of adults who received the first diagnosis of ASD in two Italian university centers *(To learn the most common past diagnoses)*.

What Are the Key Findings/Results of the Article?

Five disorders (schizophrenia, psychotic disorder, bipolar disorder, major depressive disorder, and personality disorder) were specifically highlighted as misdiagnosed psychiatric diseases or comorbidities responsible for unrecognized ASD. The most common past diagnoses were intellectual disability, psychosis, personality disorders, and depression.

What are the Implications for Future Projects Identified by Authors (Creating a Need)?

Other than diagnostic problems, clinicians should pay more attention to the association between their functioning, adjustment, and mental health beyond symptomatology. For better mental health and social adjustment in patients with ASD, correct diagnosis of ASD, treatments of psychiatric comorbidity, and improvements in functioning and adjustment are comprehensively necessary.

- That individuals with ASD may remain unrecognized until social demands exceed their socio-communication capacities, causing severe distress that may lead to a psychiatric consultation or hospitalization, given the overlapping symptoms with

- Other disorders, and the high rates of psychiatric co-occurrent conditions in people with ASD, it is important to consider the possibility of an ASD diagnosis in adults who are referred to mental health services.

Next Step: Literature-Supported Next Steps

What Were the Implications for the Future Identified?

1. For better mental health and social adjustment in patients with ASD, correct diagnosis of ASD, treatments of psychiatric comorbidity, and improvements in functioning and adjustment are comprehensively necessary (Takara et al., 2015).
2. Individuals with ASD may remain unrecognized until social demands exceed their socio-communication capacities, causing severe distress (Fusar-Poli et al., 2022).
3. Consider the possibility of an ASD diagnosis in adults who are referred to mental health services (Fusar-Poli et al., 2022).

Next Step: Relevance to OT

1. OTs evaluate and treat for improvements in functioning and adjustment;
2. OTs evaluate and treat for improvements in social demands and socio-communication;
3. OTs work with adults referred to mental health services;
4. OTs work on multidisciplinary teams.

Next Step: Explicitly Link the Relevance to Occupational Therapy and Expand the Literature Review

1. Occupational therapists' expertise in evaluation and treating individuals' functional abilities (AKA occupational performance) could improve accuracy of ASD diagnosis and improve the mental health and social adjustment for individuals diagnosed with ASD. NEXT: Expanded literature search terms – evaluation of functional abilities and ASD; treatment of functional abilities and ASD.
2. Occupational therapists' expertise in evaluation and treating individuals' social demands and socio-communication (AKA communication and social participation) could improve accuracy of ASD diagnosis and improve the mental health and social adjustment for individuals diagnosed with ASD. NEXT: Expanded literature search terms – evaluation of social demands and socio-communication and ASD; treatment of social demands and socio-communication and ASD.
3. Occupational therapists evaluate and treat adults referred to mental health services who may be undiagnosed with ASD. Occupational therapists' expertise in evaluation and treating adults referred to mental health services could improve accuracy of ASD diagnosis and improve the mental health and social adjustment for this population. NEXT: Expanded search terms – occupational therapy evaluation of adults receiving mental health services; occupational therapy treatment of adults receiving mental health services.

Worksheet 3.1: Selecting a Relevant Problem from the Literature

Purpose: This Worksheet Will Help You Organize Your Literature so You Can:

1. Identify the problem that the larger community of experts is currently addressing;
2. Identify what is known about the phenomena;
3. Plan how occupational therapy is the profession to address the problem OR how the profession of occupational therapy can best approach the problem.

After you have spent some time in the literature, pick your favorite three articles that address your area of interest.

If you are using a literature grid, these are the three columns you will be focused on.

Table 3.2 Three Columns of Focus

What questions did the author answer?	What are the key findings/ results or summary of the article	What are the implications for future research identified by authors (creating a need)?

What Questions Did the Author Answer?

Summarize the problems that were addressed by the subject matter experts writing about the population you are interested in. Re-read the questions answered. Reading the title of the article tends to provide guidance on what the larger problem that is trying to be solved is.

If more than one author is addressing the same problem/asking the same questions, cite the multiple authors in the left-hand column of the table below. If more authors are researching a topic, that makes your project objectives stronger.

Table 3.3 Top Three Questions/Problems Being Addressed

Author(s)	Top three questions/problems being addressed by the authors you have read
	1
	2
	3

What Are the Key Findings/Results of What the Author Reported on After Completing Their Study?

Summarize the findings that were addressed by the subject matter experts writing about the population you are interested in. Re-read the discussion section of the article – this tends to be the section that restates the most important aspects of the findings.

If more than one author has similar findings/results, cite the multiple authors in the left-hand column of the table below. If more authors are researching a topic, that makes your project objectives stronger.

Table 3.4 Top Three Findings/Results Being Addressed

Author(s)	Top three findings/results being addressed by the authors you have read
	1
	2
	3

What Are the Implications for the Future Stated by the Author?

Summarize the implications for the future that were addressed by the subject matter experts writing about the population you are interested in. Re-read the future implications or summary section of the article.

If more than one author has stated similar implications for the future, cite the multiple authors in the left-hand column of the table below. If more authors are researching a topic, that makes your project objectives stronger.

Table 3.5 Top Three Implications for the Future

Author (s)	Top three implications for the future being addressed by the authors you have read
	1
	2
	3

What Are the Implications for Occupational Therapy?

Summarize the implications for occupational therapy by looking at the implications for the future (see above) and linking them to the profession. If the literature states that an occupational therapist could do something in the future, write these options in the table below. If the literature states something should be done, but doesn't directly state occupational therapists should fill this gap, can you find an article that states occupational therapists could fill the gap?

Table 3.6 Top Three Implications for Occupational Therapy

Author(s)	Top three implications for occupational therapy
	1
	2
	3

Review the Top Three Implications for Occupational Therapy. Which of the Following Categories Align with Your Findings?

Since the goal of the capstone is to develop a project and have an experience where you have in-depth exposure, it is common to have a primary category for the project and then develop objectives for multiple categories for the experience.

Table 3.7 Categories for the Project

Clinical practice skills	Administration	Program and policy development	Education
Research skills	Leadership	Advocacy	Theory development

From the categories identified:

1. What category do you think your project type will be?
2. What categories might you create and have exposure to during the experience?

What to Do When You're Feeling Anxious or Confused

1. Having a peer partner can be of great assistance. They are someone who is experiencing the same journey and can help you in clearly articulating your ideas and meeting academic requirements. In addition, it is advisable to create a concept map or something comparable to visually illustrate your argument and provide evidence.
2. Think long-term. The objective is to emphasize that the learning process does not end when a project is selected. During the development of the capstone project, it is essential to continue learning, solicit feedback, and ensure you are communicating accurately.
3. Take a break. Things that are important to you can cause confusion, stress, or anxiety. If it wasn't important to you, you wouldn't be having these feelings. Congratulate yourself that you are trying to help to solve a larger problem and that you are actively recognizing how you can contribute to better the world!

TIPS

Read Research Articles that Are Less than Three Years Old

When carrying out a literature review, be as comprehensive as possible. Knowing exactly where to get information is critical. Differentiate types of articles in scholarly journals. You might get advice from your professor on which scholarly articles to use so as to be confident in your selection.

Is There a Need To Read Entire Articles Considering that Some of Them Are Very Long?

Not all the time! In the beginning of the process, reading the abstract, the findings, and the implications for the future will serve to narrow down the problem. However, as you prepare to develop the specifics of your project, take the time to read entire articles to learn how other researchers have developed their programs and research projects.

Which Areas Should I Focus on While Reading Literature?

When conducting a literature review, sometimes the gaps will be stated clearly. Other times you may need to take note of where the gaps are in the conversation, as well as what the study has covered so far, the methods used, and how a different approach to the problem might result in a different outcome. You should pay attention to these key areas:

- The posed research question;
- The theories being applied, critiqued, or tested – and why;
- The study's limitations – this is where the author might write exactly what could be done differently;
- Data analysis methods;
- Suggestions for the future. If the authors wrote suggestions, this is a clear direction for an OTD project.

REFERENCES

Fusar-Poli, L., Brondino, N., Politi, P., & Aguglia, E. (2022). Missed Diagnoses and Misdiagnoses of Adults with Autism Spectrum Disorder. European *Archives of Psychiatry and Clinical Neuroscience, 272*(2), 187–198.

Garrard, J. (2022). *Health Sciences Literature Review Made Easy: The Matrix Method.* Jones & Bartlett Learning.

Takara, K., Kondo, T., & Kuba, T. (2015). How and Why Is Autism Spectrum Disorder Misdiagnosed In Adult Patients?: From Diagnostic Problem to Management for Adjustment. *Mental Health in Family Medicine, 11*(2), 73–88.

Zimmer, M., Desch, L., Rosen, L. D., Bailey, M. L., & Wiley, S. E. (2012). Sensory Integration Therapies for Children with Developmental and Behavioral Disorders. *Pediatrics, 129*(6), 1186–1189.

4

What Is the Capstone Project Purpose?
Alignment of the Problem to the Project Type

Identifying a current, relevant problem is only the first step in a capstone project; the real magic occurs when the problem is effectively addressed through the lens of an occupational therapist. After reviewing the literature, you begin to understand what is being done to improve on the problem. Initially, as an occupational therapist, you recognize a general issue or occupational challenge faced by a client, such as difficulty in performing daily activities due to a recent injury.

This is an important first step, similar to selecting a broad area of focus for your capstone project. The real skill, however, lies in delving deeper to understand the specific nuances of the client's condition and occupational deficits. In occupational therapy, you conduct assessments and observe the client to pinpoint the exact areas of difficulty; for a capstone, you review literature, and seek mentorship to refine the focus of your capstone project. As you frame your intervention by theoretical model(s), an evidence-based approach emerges.

LET'S APPLY THIS CONCEPT TOWARDS THE CAPSTONE PROJECT TYPES

If an identified problem, found in the implications section of many research articles, is a lack of services addressing it, the capstone project type that best aligns with this problem is a program and policy development capstone project.

Your project type needs to directly address the identified problem. Assuring this alignment between the problem and purpose increases the likelihood that you make a real change to improve the situation.

LET'S LOOK AT A FEW EXAMPLES
Problem Statement

The problem is there are *limited services* for parents of adolescents with developmental disabilities during the transition into adulthood that address occupational performance by promoting self-efficacy on adolescents' post-secondary outcomes (Ho et al., 2023; Kirby et al., 2020).

Purpose Statement 1 (Lacks Alignment)

The purpose of this *research*-type capstone for parents of adolescents with developmental disabilities during the transition into adulthood that address occupational performance by promoting self-efficacy on adolescents' post-secondary outcomes (Ho et al., 2023; Kirby et al., 2020).

Purpose Statement 2 (Aligned)

The purpose of this *program development*-type capstone for parents of adolescents with developmental disabilities during the transition into adulthood that address occupational performance by promoting self-efficacy on adolescents' post-secondary outcomes (Ho et al., 2023; Kirby et al., 2020).

If you found the following problem identified in the literature, which project type should be identified in your purpose statement?

Matching Options

a. Research-Type Project
b. Program and Policy Development-Type Project
c. Clinical Practice Skills Project
d. Administration Project
e. Leadership Project
f. Advocacy Project
g. Education Project

Table 4.1 Matching Problem Options to Project Type

1. There is a need to solve issues within organizational management, a process optimization, or administrative system.
2. There is a need to address educational challenges, develop new teaching methodologies, or improve a learning experience for a group or population.
3. There is a lack of understanding or unexplored areas in a specific field of study.
4. There is a need to enhance leadership skills, strategies, or address leadership-related issues in an organization.
5. There is a need to design or improve a program to address a particular need or issue.
6. There is a need to advocate between or for a particular group, cause, or policy, to bring about improved communication, social or political change.
7. There is a need to enhance or develop new clinical methodologies, systems, or practices in a healthcare setting.

Answers: 1. d, 2. g, 3. a, 4. e, 5. f, 6. b, 7. c

Worksheet 4.1: Developing a Purpose Statement

Step 1

Select 3–5 articles that align with your area of focus:

Table 4.2 3–5 Articles that Align with Your Area of Focus

Article 1

Article 2

Article 3

Article 4

Article 5

Step 2

Collect the implications suggested for the future from the articles selected (column 4 if you are using the Literature Review Grid).

Table 4.3 Implications for the Future

	Implications/suggestions for the future
Article 1	

Article 2

Article 3

Article 4

Article 5

Step 3

Using the categories provided by your academic institution, identify common themes about what should be done in the future.

Potential options: clinical practice skills, research skills, administration, leadership, program and policy development, advocacy, education

Table 4.4 Identify Common Themes

	What are the implications for the future identified by authors (creating a need)?
Article 1	

Article 2

Article 3

Article 4

Article 5

Step 4

Write your draft problem statement here:

Step 5

Draft two purpose statements that align with the literature and the problem statement.

Use this as a guide: 'The purpose of this (pick one: clinical practice skills, research skills, administration, leadership, program and policy development, advocacy, education)-type capstone project is to (pick the one that aligns: develop a program; qual research = explore, quant = analyze; advocate to) _____
____'

Table 4.5 Purpose Statements

Purpose statement 1

Purpose statement 2

Step 6

Align the problem and purpose statements.

Table 4.6 Edited Purpose Statements

Edited problem statement
Edited purpose statement 1
Edited purpose statement 2

Step 7

Which of the two purpose statements interests you the most?

Worksheet 4.1 Example: Developing a Purpose Statement

Sample Process for Finding an Evidence-Informed Project Type

Area of interest: occupational therapy and concussion
    The capstone project types: clinical practice skills, research skills, administration, leadership, program and policy development, advocacy, education.

Step 1

Select 3–5 articles that align with your area of focus:
    Refer to the Literature Review Grid at the end of Chapter 4.

Table 4.7 Example of 3–5 Articles that Align with Your Area of Focus

Article 1 (Qual): Roelke, M. B., Jewell, V. D., & Radomski, M. V. (2022). Return-to-activity: Exploration of Occupational Therapy in Outpatient Adult Concussion Rehabilitation. *OTJR: Occupation, Participation and Health, 42*(4), 333–343. https://doi.org/10.1177/15394492221108649.

Article 2 (Quant): Martini, D. N., Wilhelm, J., Lee, L., Brumbach, B. H., Chesnutt, J., Skorseth, P., & King, L. A. (2022). Exploring Age and Sex Patterns for Rehabilitation Referrals after a Concussion: A Retrospective Analysis. *Archives of Rehabilitation Research and Clinical Translation, 4*(2), 100183. https://doi.org/10.1016/j.arrct.2022.100183.

Article 3 (Quant): Mathews, A., Banubakode, S., Hughes, J., Wright, B., Nagele, M., Waris, Y., & Junegst, S. (2022). Factors Associated with Receiving Inpatient Rehabilitation after Traumatic Brain Injury in a County Hospital System. *Archives of Physical Medicine and Rehabilitation, 103*(12). https://doi.org/10.1016/j.apmr.2022.08.632.

Article 1 (Qual): Roelke, M. B., Jewell, V. D., & Radomski, M. V. (2022). Return-to-activity: Exploration of Occupational Therapy in Outpatient Adult Concussion Rehabilitation. *OTJR: Occupation, Participation and Health*, *42*(4), 333–343. https://doi.org/10.1177/15394492221108649.

Article 4 (Quant): Harris, M. B., Rafeedie, S., McArthur, D., Babikian, T., Snyder, A., Polster, D., & Giza, C. C. (2019). Addition of Occupational Therapy to an Interdisciplinary Concussion Clinic Improves Identification of Functional Impairments. *The Journal of Head Trauma Rehabilitation*, *34*(6), 425–432.

Article 5

Step 2

Collect the implications suggested for the future from the articles selected (Column 4 if you are using the Literature Review Grid).

Table 4.8 Example of Implications for the Future

	Implications/suggestions for the future
Article 1: *Roelke, Jewell, & Radomski (2022)*	*TIP: Found in the abstract:* 'Further research is needed to develop best practices for concussion rehabilitation from acute to chronic symptoms, symptom profile evaluation and interventions, their efficacy, and return-to-activity outcomes.' *TIP: Found in the implications for clinical practice and future research:* 'The logic model guides practitioners through essential process and outcome domains, including specific expert-endorsed evaluation and intervention tools. It provides a framework for practitioners to advocate for participation in concussion rehabilitation programs, particularly sports CPs and policy planning. Further research is needed to develop best practices for concussion rehabilitation from acute to chronic symptoms, symptom profile evaluation and interventions, their efficacy, and return-to-activity outcomes.'
Article 2: *Martini, Wilhelm, Lee, Brumbach, Chesnutt, Skorseth, & King (2022)*	*TIP: Found in the abstract:* 'Improving concussion education dissemination across all entry points of a level 1 trauma center may standardize the postconcussion rehabilitation referral patterns, potentially improving the time to recovery from a concussion.' *TIP: Found in the conclusion:* 'highlights the need for streamlined post-concussion care, increasing the dissemination of standardized concussion education materials to medical professionals across all disciplines may reduce the variability of post-concussion care patterns. More work is needed on prospectively following patients through the recovery process to determine the most efficacious post-concussion care for any age, sex, and preexisting comorbidity.'

45

	Implications/suggestions for the future
Article 3: *Mathews, Banuba-kode, Hughes, Wright, Nagele, Waris, & Junegst (2022)*	*TIP: Found in the abstract:* 'Future research should assess potential reasons for these differences and work to improve access to rehabilitation after TBI.' *TIP: Found in the conclusion:* 'In our study, similar to prior research, factors like insurance status, race, primary language spoken, and injury severity differed between patients that did versus those that did not receive inpatient rehabilitation. Future research should assess potential reasons for these differences and work to improve access to rehabilitation after TBI.'
Article 4: *Harris, Rafeedie, McArthur, Babikian, Snyder, Polster, & Giza (2019)*	*TIP: Found in the future directions:* 'Currently, there is limited research identifying the need for an occupational therapy practitioner's role in a concussion clinic.' *TIP: Found in the conclusion:* 'This study demonstrates that a greater number of impacted domains were identified and reported when an OT completed an assessment during a joint evaluation of chronic patients recovering from traumatic brain injury, rather than when assessed by a physician alone. Occupational therapy practitioners can provide a unique contribution to the plan of care, with a variety of evidence-based interventions and occupation-based domains that are beneficial to this patient population.'
Article 5	

Step 3

Using the categories provided by your academic institution, identify common themes about what should be done in the future.

Options: **clinical practice skills**, *research skills*, administration, leadership, **program and policy development**, ADVOCACY, EDUCATION.

Table 4.9 Example of Identifying Common Themes

	What are the implications for the future identified by authors (creating a need)?
Article 1	'Further *research* is needed to **develop best practices** for concussion rehabilitation from acute to chronic symptoms, **symptom profile evaluation and interventions**, their efficacy, and return-to-activity outcomes.'
Article 2	'Improving concussion EDUCATION dissemination across all entry points of a level 1 trauma center may standardize the post-concussion rehabilitation referral patterns, potentially improving the time to recovery from a concussion.' 'highlights the need for **streamlined post-concussion care**, increasing the dissemination of standardized concussion EDUCATION materials to medical professionals across all disciplines may reduce the variability of post-concussion care patterns. More work is needed on *prospectively* following patients through the recovery process to determine the most efficacious post-concussion care for any age, sex, and preexisting comorbidity.'

Article 3	'*Future research* should assess potential reasons for THESE DIFFERENCES and work to **improve access to rehabilitation after TBI**.'
Article 4	'Currently, there is *limited research* identifying the need for an **occupational therapy practitioner's role in a concussion clinic**.' 'This study demonstrates that a greater number of impacted domains were identified and reported when an OT **completed an assessment during** a joint evaluation of chronic patients recovering from traumatic brain injury, rather than when assessed by a physician alone. Occupational therapy practitioners can provide a unique contribution to the plan of care, with a variety of **evidence-based interventions** and occupation-based domains that are beneficial to this patient population.'

Step 4

Write your draft problem statement here:

   The problem is there is limited research identifying the need for occupational therapists on an interdisciplinary concussion team to help improve impacted areas of daily life and performance (Harris et al., 2019; Martini et al., 2022).

Step 5

Draft two purpose statements that align with the literature and the problem statement.

   Use this as a guide: 'The purpose of this (pick one: clinical practice skills, research skills, administration, leadership, program and policy development, advocacy, education)-type capstone project is to (pick the one that aligns: develop a program; qual research = explore, quant = analyze; advocate to) _____'

Table 4.10 Example of Purpose Statements

Purpose statement 1:
The purpose of this program and policy development capstone project is to develop and implement a program for individuals with mTBI or post-concussion syndrome, to provide occupational therapy evaluation and intervention to improve impacted areas of daily life and performance for the population.

Purpose statement 2
The purpose of this research-type capstone project is to explore (qual) occupational therapist evaluation and intervention on a concussion team to fill the gap in the literature about best practices of OTs on the concussion team.

Step 6

Align the problem and purpose statements.

Table 4.11 Example of Edited Purpose Statements

Edited problem statement:
The problem is a lack of programs for occupational therapists to evaluate and treat individuals with post-concussion syndrome resulting in fewer OTs practicing on the interdisciplinary team (Harris et al., 2019; Roelke et al., 2022).
The problem is there is limited research identifying the need for occupational therapists on an interdisciplinary concussion team to develop best practices for the profession (Harris et al., 2019; Martini et al., 2022).

Edited purpose statement 1:
The purpose of this program and policy development capstone project is to develop and implement a program for occupational therapists to evaluate and treat individuals with post-concussion syndrome.

Edited purpose statement 2:
The purpose of this research-type capstone project is to explore (qual) occupational therapist evaluation and intervention on a concussion team to fill the gap in the literature about best practices of OTs on the concussion team.

FOOD FOR THOUGHT

The project type can change depending on the literature you read. Below are articles that deepen the understanding of the role of occupational therapists in post-concussion care. These articles could be used to support a capstone project in each of the project types.

1. *Clinical practice skills*: Article one supports a project on clinical practice skills for occupational therapists – specifically, evaluation and intervention for individuals with mTBI/post-concussion along the continuum of care. Articles two and three support clinical practice skills of referral and interdisciplinary services for individuals with post-concussion syndrome.

Other references that support clinical practice capstone projects:

Acord-Vira, A., Davis, D., & Lilly, C. (2021). Occupational Performance Limitations After Concussion in College Students. *The American Journal of Occupational Therapy, 75*(5). https://doi.org/10.5014/ajot.2021.043398.
Acord-Vira, A., & Davis, D. (2020). Occupational Performance Limitations Experienced by Postsecondary Students Following Concussion. *The American Journal of Occupational*

Therapy, *74*(4, Supplement_1), 7411510337p1–7411510337p1. https://doi.org/10.5014/ajot.2020.74s1-rp304b.

Harris, M. B., Rafeedie, S., McArthur, D., Babikian, T., Snyder, A., Polster, D., & Giza, C. C. (2019). Addition of Occupational Therapy to an Interdisciplinary Concussion Clinic Improves Identification Of Functional Impairments. *Journal of Head Trauma Rehabilitation*, *34*(6), 425–432. https://doi.org/10.1097/htr.0000000000000544.

Opinion: AOTA: Managing Concussion: Occupational Therapy's Role in Evaluating and Treating Athletes (2021). Aota.org. https://www.aota.org/publications-news/otp/archive/2021/managing-concussion.aspx.

2. *Research skills*: All articles listed above explicitly support research-type projects.
3. *Administration*: Combining the recommendations of all the articles supports a project focused on the administrative practices of: referral to rehabilitation, OT evaluation, OT intervention for individuals who are post-concussion.

   Other options would be to look at literature that would support the administrative aspects of referrals for individuals for follow-up after a concussion. Use search terms such as healthcare administration, referrals, healthcare systems, and concussion. The following are sources that could be used:

   Zayoud, M. (2023). Healthcare System. In *Process Mining Techniques for Managing and Improving Healthcare Systems*. CRC Press, pp. 1–12. https://doi.org/10.1201/9781003366577-1.

   Agnihotri, S., Penner, M., Mallory, K. D., Xie, L., Hickling, A., Joachimides, N., Widgett, E., & Scratch, S. E. (2021). Healthcare Utilization and Costs Associated with Persistent Post-Concussive Symptoms. *Brain Injury*, *35*(11), 1382–1389. https://doi.org/10.1080/02699052.2021.1972151.

   Karatas, M., Eriskin, L., Deveci, M., Pamucar, D., & Garg, H. (2022). Big Data for Healthcare Industry 4.0: Applications, Challenges and Future Perspectives. *Expert Systems with Applications*, *200*, 116912. https://doi.org/10.1016/j.eswa.2022.116912.

   Marshall, S., & van Ierssel, J. (2022). Management of Concussion and Persistent Post-Concussion Symptoms. In: T. A. Schweizer & A. J. Baker (eds.), *Tackling the Concussion Epidemic*. Springer, pp. 153–180. https://doi.org/10.1007/978-3-030-93813-0_8.

4. *Leadership*: Combining the recommendations of all the above articles supports a project focused on the leadership practices of: occupational therapists to serve individuals who are post-concussion, leadership practices of different disciplines to provide appropriate and timely referral.

   Jennings, T., & Islam, M. S. (2022). Examining the Interdisciplinary Approach for Treatment of Persistent Post-Concussion Symptoms in Adults: A Systematic Review. *Brain Impairment*, 1–19. https://doi.org/10.1017/brimp.2022.28.

   Marshall, S., & van Ierssel, J. (2022). Management of Concussion and Persistent Post-Concussion Symptoms. In: T. A. Schweizer & A. J. Baker (eds.), *Tackling the Concussion Epidemic*. Springer, pp. 153–180. https://doi.org/10.1007/978-3-030-93813-0_8.

5. *For consideration*: Theory development. Although at first glance these articles do not support a theory development-type capstone.

   Anderson, B. R. (2017). Improving Health Care by Embracing Systems Theory. *The Journal of Thoracic and Cardiovascular Surgery*, *152*(2), 593–594. https://doi.org/10.1016/j.jtcvs.2016.03.029.

WHICH ONE INTERESTS YOU THE MOST?

1. How do I know the problem or issue identified in my literature review matches with the purpose or goal of my capstone project?

   Answer: To ensure alignment, define the problem clearly supported by the literature. Select a type of capstone project that addresses this issue directly. If a knowledge gap is identified in the literature review, for instance, a project of the research variety would be suitable. To ensure alignment, consistently refer back to the problem throughout the duration of the project.

2. How do I determine which project type is best when the literature review identifies several potential project types?

Answer: When the literature review identifies multiple feasible project types, consider the following to pick one:

a. Select a project type that matches your areas of expertise and personal interests. This will help you maintain motivation and engagement throughout the project. In other words: Pick the project type that is most interesting to you!

b. Look at your available resources, including but not limited to time, mentorship, and availability of experiential sites. These factors will influence which project types are more feasible than others.

c. Consider which category of project could have the most substantial outcomes towards improving the identified issue. Which project type could have the greatest contribution to the profession or the population?

3. Can my capstone project type address more than one type?

Answer: The short answer is: Does your institution allow students to do more than one capstone project? Although it is feasible to tackle more than one issue during the capstone experience, for the project, try to maintain a concentrated approach. For clarity and depth, your capstone project should primarily address one central problem and project type.

Other articles to get from the references of the articles reviewed:

Table 4.13 Other Articles

REFERENCES

American Occupational Therapy Association (2020). Occupational Therapy Practice Framework: Domain and Process – Fourth Edition. *American Journal of Occupational Therapy*, *74*(sup_2), 7412410010. https://doi.org/10.5014/ajot.2020.74S2001.

Eco, U. (2015). *How to Write a Thesis*. MIT Press.

Ho, Y. R., Chen, B. Y., & Li, C. M. (2023). Thinking More Wisely: Using the Socratic Method to Develop Critical Thinking Skills Amongst Healthcare Students. *BMC Medical Education*, *23*(1), 173.

Kirby, A. V., Feldman, K. J. C., Hoffman, J. M., Diener, M. L., & Himle, M. B. (2020). Transition Preparation Activities and Expectations for the Transition to Adulthood Among Parents of Autistic Youth. *Research in Autism Spectrum Disorders*, *78*, 101640.

Selvia, A. (2020). A Socratic Teaching Method to Foster Critical Thinking Skills among Nursing Students in Our Clinical Classroom Settings. *South Asian Research Journal of Nursing and Healthcare*, *2*(4), 1–11.

Literature Review Grid

Purpose: Use the sections in this grid to organize the literature you read. Each column has a different purpose in the development of your capstone.

Procedures: If possible, cut and paste the information from the articles into the grid.

Comments: The literature review grid is a working document. There are articles that will be included while you are learning about a population or a problem that will be deleted due to redundancy or changing direction of the project.

Suggestions: 1) one page per article, 2) Change the font size of the header to 10 pt font as it takes up less space on the page.

Student name: OTD Student

Title of capstone project: I don't know yet. My area of interest is the neurological population, specifically mTBI and concussion

Databases used: Google Scholar

Key words: Concussion, Rehabilitation, Occupational Therapy

Table 4.12 Literature Review Grid

1	2	3	4	5	6	7
Article citation in APA	What questions did the author answer?	What are the key findings/ summary of the article	What are the implications for the future identified by authors (creating a need)	Overall evaluation of the article in relation to your capstone Analyze how the article relates to your capstone project. What are the top 2–3 pieces of information from this article that could be used in your capstone? Putting this in your own words will help you when writing later.	What type of study is this? Include: a variety but a minimum of: 3 quantitative 3 qualitative 1 systematic review or meta-analysis 1 book 1 international study	Did this article support: Purpose Problem Background Significance This section will help you pull relevant articles when writing each section. Look for common themes and identify them.

(Continued)

Table 4.12 (Continued)

1	2	3	4	5	6	7
1. Roelke, M. B., Jewell, V. D., & Radomski, M. V. (2022). Return-to-activity: Exploration of Occupational Therapy in Outpatient Adult Concussion Rehabilitation. *OTJR: Occupation, Participation and Health, 42*(4), 333–343. https://doi.org/10.1177/15394492221108649.	*TIP: Found in the abstract:* 'describe the occupational therapy process of evaluation and intervention for adults with a history of concussion(s) and persisting symptoms.'	*TIP: Found in the abstract:* 'a description of how occupational therapy practitioners, across practice settings, aid individuals in returning to everyday activities and life roles after concussion(s).' *Another option that could be helpful (menu option #9):* 'Content analysis with a deductive strategy, open coding, and an unconstrained matrix was used to determine the process portion of a logic model outlining how expert practitioners framed their approach to rehabilitation.'	*TIP: Implications for clinical practice and future research:* 'Further research is needed to develop best practices for concussion rehabilitation from acute to chronic symptoms, symptom profile evaluation and interventions, their efficacy, and return-to-activity outcomes.'	*TIP: Found in the conclusion:* 'describes preliminary specifications regarding what constitutes best practices for occupational therapy practitioners in concussion rehabilitation' Knowing this information will be helpful to learn what OTs do with this population.	*TIP: Found in the abstract:* Qualitative: *Another option that could be helpful (menu option #10):* 'qualitative descriptive study used focus groups of expert occupational therapy practitioners across practice settings.'	Problem

52

2. Martini, D. N., Wilhelm, J., Lee, L., Brumbach, B. H. Chesnutt, J., Skorseth, P, & King, L. A. (2022). Exploring Age and Sex Patterns for Rehabilitation Referrals after a Concussion: A Retrospective Analysis. *Archives of Rehabilitation Research and Clinical Translation, 4*(2), 100183. https://doi.org/10.1016/.arrct.2022.100183.

TIP: Found in the abstract: 'To explore patterns of postconcussion care at a level 1 trauma center.'

TIP: Found in the abstract: 'Point of entry, age, sex, and preexisting comorbidities are associated with postconcussion care rehabilitation referral patterns.'

TIP: Found in the abstract: 'Improving concussion education dissemination across all entry points of a level 1 trauma center may standardize the postconcussion rehabilitation referral patterns, potentially improving the time to recovery from a concussion.'

TIP: Found in the conclusion: 'highlights the need for streamlined postconcussion care. Increasing the dissemination of standardized concussion education materials to medical professionals across all disciplines may reduce the variability of postconcussion care patterns. More work is needed on prospectively following patients through the recovery process to determine the most efficacious postconcussion care for any age, sex, and preexisting comorbidity.'

TIP: Found in the conclusion: 'rehabilitation referrals may decrease recovery time and address important preexisting comorbidities that may otherwise be overlooked during the postconcussion care visit. There is significant variability in postconcussion care, particularly for older adults where the guidelines are not clear. Point of entry into the medical system appears to affect postconcussion care.'

Problem

TIP: Found in the abstract: Qualitative
Another option that could be helpful (menu option #9): Level of evidence = Level II – Retrospective study
N= 2417

54

Table 4.12 (Continued)

1	2	3	4	5	6	7
3. Mathews, A., Banubakode, S., Hughes, J., Wright, B., Nagele, M., Waris, Y., & Junegst, S. (2022). Factors Associated with Receiving Inpatient Rehabilitation after Traumatic Brain Injury in a County Hospital System. *Archives of Physical Medicine and Rehabilitation, 103*(12). https://doi.org/10.1016/j.apmr.2022.08.632.	*TIP: Found in the abstract:* 'To characterize factors associated with inpatient rehabilitation for individuals with Traumatic Brain Injury (TBI) presenting to an Emergency Department (ED) at a local county hospital.'	*TIP: Found in the abstract:* 'similar to prior research, factors like insurance status, race, primary language spoken, and injury severity differed between patients that did versus those that did not receive inpatient rehabilitation.'	*TIP: Found in the abstract:* 'Future research should assess potential reasons for these differences and work to improve access to rehabilitation after TBI.'	*TIP: Found in the abstract:* This study identified a TBI Model System. When I went to learn what model that is, I found a national database that I will look at later. 'Inpatient rehabilitation (Yes/No) after moderate-severe TBI as defined by the TBI Model Systems criteria (trauma-related imaging abnormalities, loss of consciousness >30 minutes, post-traumatic amnesia >24 hours, and/or Glasgow Coma Scale score < 13).'	*TIP: Found in the abstract:* Qualitative *Another option that could be helpful (menu option #9):* Level of evidence = Level II – Retrospective study N= 152	Problem

5

Finding a Problem and Writing a Problem Statement

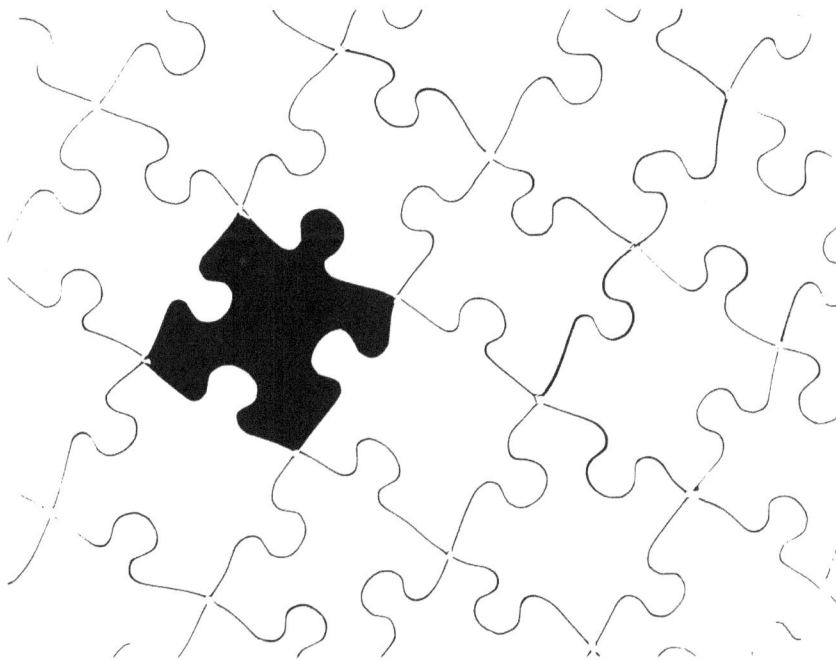

Figure 5.1 Piece of a Puzzle

WHAT'S YOUR PROBLEM?

A problem statement is a concise description of an issue that needs to be improved upon. The problem statement identifies a gap between a specific, current issue (problem) and a desired process or outcome (the goal). The problem statement is necessary to give a clear and specific statement of the problem, which helps to narrow down the project's goals and scope.

Before writing a problem statement, you should read and organize existing literature to learn what other people working in the field consider the issues and causes of the issues to be. You did this in Chapter 4 when you selected a minimum number of articles to read from different categories. Once you start to understand the problem, create an initial problem statement. A well-defined problem statement helps in setting the direction for your project. It serves as a guide to keep the project focused and defines the goals and objectives that need to be achieved. This clarity allows your doctoral coordinator(s), mentors, and supervisors to better support your project and guide the experience.

A clear problem statement also helps the project stay on track by narrowing the goals and objectives that will be the focus of the project.

FINDING A PROBLEM AND WRITING A PROBLEM STATEMENT IS A PROCESS, NOT A TASK

The process of finding a problem and writing a problem statement is not a one-time thing that you do. The problem statement will continue to develop as you read more literature, learn from mentors, and deepen your understanding of the problem. This iterative method makes sure that the problem is correctly identified and clearly stated, changing as new information and insights are gained.

As occupational therapy students, you have the opportunity to select an area of interest to complete a project and have an experience to understand how occupational therapy can improve a problem and how it best supports people's lives. However, as a student you have a limited amount of time to complete the project and experience, and you will need to narrow your problem down by creating objectives that are achievable within a certain time frame.

MULTIFACETED PURPOSES OF A PROBLEM STATEMENT

The problem statement clarifies the project's scope, goals, and relationship to the profession of occupational therapy. As the project develops, the problem statement acts as a navigator for this project. It will be referred back to during the duration of the project in order to help you to remain on track and focused.

For the First Draft of a Problem Statement:

A first draft is to guide your creative thinking and strategic planning
    Keep it short:
    The problem is_____ which results in_____
    Make sure the problem is relevant to the profession.
    Discuss the problem with faculty, mentors, and learn as much as you can about what is known about the problem.
    The problem statement will change, and keep changing, as you learn more.

USE THE LITERATURE REVIEW GRID TO IDENTIFY AND DEFEND THE PROBLEM

In Chapter 4, you selected relevant articles and gathered essential information from them. This step was crucial for beginning to comprehend the existing literature that underpins your understanding of a particular issue. This foundational work is instrumental in building a solid knowledge base about the topic you are exploring.

If you begin to track the literature you read early and often, the process of writing a literature review will be easier. You can start by using a reference management system like Zotero or Mendeley (there are others), or use a literature grid like the one above.

The purpose of this grid is to use the sections in it to organize the literature you read. Each column has a different purpose in the development of your capstone. The benefit of using a grid versus saving each article is that you input information in each category, so you can remember which article reported specific topics. Note: the grid in Table 5.1 offers suggestions on what to include and each column is discussed in more depth in Chapter 10, 'Literature Review'.

Table 5.1 Literature Review Grid Columns

1	2	3	4	5	6	7
Article citation in APA	What questions did the author answer?	What are the key findings/ summary of the article	What are the implications for the future identified by authors (creating a need)?	Overall evaluation of the article in relation to your capstone Analyze how the article relates to your capstone project. What are the top 2–3 pieces of information from this article that could be used in your capstone? Putting this in your own words will help you when writing later.	What type of study is this? Include a variety but a minimum of: 3 quantitative 3 qualitative 1 systematic review or meta-analysis 1 book 1 international study	Did this article support: Purpose Problem Background Significance? This section will help you pull relevant articles when writing each section. Look for common themes and identify them.

WHAT IS ENOUGH LITERATURE TO DRAFT A PROBLEM STATEMENT?

The short answer is there should be at least two current (from less than 3–5 years ago) research-type articles that support that there is a specific problem. It is challenging to figure out which key terms to focus on when you begin reading literature. As you start exploring an area of interest, read the abstract and the conclusion. Focusing on just these aspects allows you to see the breadth of an area of interest. When you feel you have read enough to understand the problem and you are ready to draft a problem statement, narrow the literature you have read to current literature, as mentioned. This ensures the focus of your problem aligns with other experts addressing the problem. Using older sources for the problem statement risks taking the problem's focus in a direction that is not relevant, or has already proven ineffective.

Worksheet 5.1: Literature Review Grid, or Identify this Information

Purpose: Use the sections in this grid to organize the literature you read. Each column has a different purpose in the development of your capstone.

As you look down column 4 – what are common themes about the work being done in your area of interest? Consider each of the authors to be your personal subject matter experts. What do these experts think needs to be done next to improve the outcomes for the population or problem you have chosen?

Table 5.2 Literature Review Grid Columns

1	2	3	4	5	6	7
Article citation in APA	What questions did the author answer?	What are the key findings/ summary of the article	What are the implications for the future identified by authors (creating a need)?	Overall evaluation of the article in relation to your capstone Analyze how the article relates to your capstone project. What are the top 2–3 pieces of information from this article that could be used in your capstone? Putting this in your own words will help you when writing later.	What type of study is this? Include: a variety but a minimum of: 3 quantitative 3 qualitative 1 systematic review or meta-analysis 1 book 1 international study	Did this article support: Purpose Problem Background Significance This section will help you pull relevant articles when writing each section. Look for common themes and identify them.

WRITING A PROBLEM STATEMENT FOR YOUR CAPSTONE PROJECT

Formulating a one- or two-sentence problem statement is a next step in determining a clear direction of the capstone project. A clear problem statement helps communicate the problem, its significance, and its relevance to your mentors, site mentors, and capstone committee in order to get approval and gain specific mentorship during the process. The problem statement places a boundary around your capstone project and guides the areas you can utilize for the capstone experience.

A well-written problem statement serves as the basis for the entire capstone project, guiding decision-making and the development of potential solutions. It is essentially a road map for the project, guiding you to identify and investigate alternatives to the capstone's demonstrated solution. For example, does the literature support developing and implementing a program (i.e., a program and policy-type capstone project), or does it support that leadership at an institution can make changes to improve the problem (i.e., a leadership-type project)? Through the capstone experience, the problem statement serves to define, clarify, and refine the problem, which facilitates effective decision-making and ultimately leads to the identification and implementation of solutions. In conclusion, for a capstone project, a carefully articulated problem statement supported by current evidence is essential for defining the problem being addressed, guiding the project's direction, and facilitating effective decision-making throughout the capstone experience. It ensures the project's relevance, encourages the exploration of multiple solutions, and facilitates a comprehensive and significant capstone undertaking.

PROCESS OF WRITING A PROBLEM STATEMENT

The process of formulating a problem statement requires careful consideration. In regards to making a decision, students are faced with the task of identifying a problem versus just selecting an area of personal interest. Choosing a personal area of interest serves as an internal drive to begin planning a capstone; however, using a personal area of interest also increases the likelihood of bias in the formation of the project. Acknowledge that as a student, you are not an expert in the area of interest. You must read literature and use faculty collaboration to understand the current issues surrounding your area of interest. Support the problem of focus on aspects identified by the literature.

Development of your problem statement is a process requiring a rigorous approach. Students can begin by writing a preliminary problem statement, with a focus on identifying existing issues and articulating how the issue can be improved through occupational therapy. Next, after the initial draft, review the statement for themes and keywords. Now you will begin reading literature to better understand the issue. As you learn more about the issue, you will develop a more precise problem statement. Time spent drafting, editing, and developing a problem statement increases the chance that your capstone project and experience will better align with your goals, and will result in a social change.

Use the worksheets in this chapter to explore the literature and draft a problem statement:

Worksheet 5.2: Developing a Problem Statement

Objective: Communicate, in writing, a clear and concise problem that is supported by current literature, and that will be improved upon by the capstone project.

Step 1: Write down the primary issue you are finding in the literature.

_____

_____

_____

_____

Step 2: Explain why this issue is happening, or the implications of this issue. Why is this an issue?

_____

_____

_____

_____

Step 3: What are two current references you have that support that a) this is an issue, and b) would agree why the issue is occurring.

_____

_____

_____

_____

Step 4: Draft these concepts into a problem statement:
The problem is _____
which results in (OR which is a problem because)

_____

_____

(Citation 1, Citation 2)

Worksheet 5.2 Example: Developing a Problem Statement

Objective: Communicate, in writing, a clear and concise problem that is supported by current literature, and that will be improved upon by the capstone project.

Step 1: Write down the primary issue you are finding in the literature.
'Individuals with dementia and their caregivers have poor health outcomes, and don't have enough support over the course of the disease progression.'

Step 2: Explain why this issue is happening, or the implications of this issue. Why is this an issue?
This is a problem because both the individual with dementia and their caregivers could have better health outcomes with more support. There are phases being identified during the progression of the disease, but there is still not enough support for this population.

Step 3: What are two current references you have that support that 1) this is an issue and 2) would agree why the issue is occurring.
Dam, A. E., de Vugt, M. E., Klinkenberg, I. P., Verhey, F. R., & van Boxtel, M. P. (2016). A Systematic Review of Social Support Interventions for Caregivers of People With Dementia: Are They Doing what They Promise?. *Maturitas, 85,* 117–130.

Kokorelias, K. M., Gignac, M. A., Naglie, G., Rittenberg, N., MacKenzie, J., D'Souza, S., & Cameron, J. I. (2022). A Grounded Theory Study to Identify Caregiving Phases and Support Needs across the Alzheimer's Disease Trajectory. *Disability and Rehabilitation, 44*(7), 1050–1059.

Step 4: Draft these concepts into a problem statement:

The problem is there aren't enough services for individuals with dementia or their caregivers to maximize daily occupational performance [which results in (OR which is a problem because)] This is a problem because individuals with dementia and their caregivers have challenges to their health and wellness, quality of life, and decreased occupational performance.

After editing here was a final problem statement:

The problem is a gap in services for post-diagnostic support for individuals diagnosed with dementia to maximize everyday functional memory performance and occupational performance (Griffin & Hope, 2022; Kwon & Kim, 2022).

Learning Activity 5.1: How Can These Problem Statements be Refined for Greater Clarity or More Directly Linked to the Profession of Occupational Therapy?

Example 1: The problem is a gap in services for post-diagnostic support for individuals diagnosed with dementia to maximize everyday functional memory performance and occupational performance (Griffin & Hope, 2022; Kwon & Kim, 2022).

Edit:

Example 2: The problem is that adults with obesity experience physical and psychosocial barriers that decrease their occupational performance and quality of life (Nossum et al., 2017; Uzogara, 2017). (Groll – student sample)

Edit:

Worksheet 5.3: Practice Drafting a Problem Statement for the Capstone Project

Examples for Each Project Type

After reading a minimum of three articles on a population or problem, which one of the following seems to be what the evidence is saying the problem is?

1. The problem is a lack of efficacy of (clinical practice skills)
2. The problem is a gap in the literature (research)
3. The problem is a lack of access to care or with process/workflow or recruitment and retention (administration)
4. The problem is lack of capacity or interprofessional collaboration (leadership)
5. The problem is a lack of services (program and policy development)
6. The problem is lack of awareness (advocacy)
7. The problem is lack of advanced training or educational resources or lack of access to training or educational resources (education)
8. The problem is decreased application of known insights (theory development).

Step 1: Answer the question: From the above list, which one or two of these problem types is supported by the implication for the future from the current literature you have read?

_____

_____

_____

Step 2: Answer the question: From the literature you read, what is the negative result that happens because of this problem?

_____

_____

_____

Step 3: Answer the question: Why is this a relevant problem for the profession of occupational therapy?

_____

_____

_____

Step 4: Write out a complete problem statement in one or two sentences with citations and references. Refer to the sample problem statements for examples as you are drafting.

The problem is

_____

_____

_____ which results in (OR which is a problem because)

_____

_____

_____

Citation 1:

Citation 2:

Worksheet 5.4: Supporting or Defending the Problem Statement

After writing a succinct problem statement, the next step will be to write a supporting paragraph or two. This section serves to deepen a reader's understanding of the value of addressing the specific issue described in the problem statement.

(Main idea sentence/topic sentence – summarize the main point of the paragraph).

Step 1: Develop the Main Idea Sentence

Sentence 1 (S1): The problem is

_____

which results in (OR which is a problem because)

_____

(Citation 1, Citation 2)

Step 2: Develop Supporting Sentences

Sentence 2 (S2): Include detail(s) that underscore the broad problem.
Sentence 3 (S3): Include detail(s) that underscore the focused problem.

Step 3: Develop a Conclusion Sentence

Summarize the purpose of the paragraph and _transition to the next paragraph or the next header_.
   EDITING NOTE: This section is generally 1–2 paragraphs.

Worksheet 5.4 Example A: Supporting or Defending the Problem Statement

Step 1: Develop the Main Idea Sentence
The problem is young adults with autism have more challenges than age-matched peers with the occupational roles of finding and keeping employment (Baker-Ericzén et al., 2022; Moody et al., 2022).

Step 2: Develop Supporting Sentences

Sentence 2 (S2): Include detail(s) that underscore the broad problem: Adults with Autism Spectrum Disorder (ASD) have access to fewer services compared to young children with ASD.
   Sentence 3 (S3): Include detail(s) that underscore the focused problem: Additionally, when transitioning out of the school system, they often lose access to services that have provided support (Baker-Ericzén et al., 2022).

Step 3: Develop a Conclusion Sentence

Summarize the purpose of the paragraph and _transition to the next paragraph or the next header_:
   Occupational therapy can address both social and communication skills for job attainment, and the work environment and person-organization fit to support employment in individuals with ASD.
   EDITING NOTE: This section is generally 1–2 paragraphs.

Step 4: Synthesize into Paragraphs

Statement of the Problem

The problem is young adults with autism have more challenges than age-matched peers with the occupational roles of finding and keeping employment. Adults with ASD receive fewer services than young children with ASD, and when leaving the school system, access to services is also lost (Turcotte et al., 2016; van Schalkwyk & Volkmar, 2017). Young adults with autism are faced with disadvantages and a lack of support in the workplace despite their willingness to work (Anderson et al., 2021). Occupational therapy can address both social and communication skills for job attainment, as noted by Rosales and Whitlow (2019), and the work environment and person-organization fit to support employment in individuals with ASD, as discussed by Hayward et al. (2019) and Hedley et al. (2018).

References

Anderson, C., Butt, C., & Sarsony, C. (2021). Young Adults on the Autism Spectrum and Early Employment-Related Experiences: Aspirations and Obstacles. *Journal of Autism and Developmental Disorders*, *51*, 88–105.

Baker-Ericzén, M. J., ElShamy, R., & Kammes, R. R. (2022). Current Status of Evidence-Based Practices to Enhance Employment Outcomes for Transition Age Youth and Adults on the Autism Spectrum. *Current Psychiatry Reports*, *24*(3), 161–170.

Hayward, S. M., McVilly, K. R., & Stokes, M. A. (2019). Autism and Employment: What Works. *Research in Autism Spectrum Disorders*, *60*, 48–58. https://doi.org/10.1016/j.rasd.2019.01.006.

Moody, C. T., Factor, R. S., Gulsrud, A. C., Grantz, C. J., Tsai, K., Jolliffe, M., Rosen, N. E., McCracken, J. T. & Laugeson, E. A. (2022). A Pilot Study of PEERS® for Careers: A Comprehensive Employment-Focused Social Skills Intervention for Autistic Young Adults in the United States. *Research in Developmental Disabilities*, *128*, 104287.

Worksheet 5.4 Example B: Supporting or Defending the Problem Statement (Groll – Student Sample)

Statement of the Problem

The problem is that adults with obesity experience physical and psychosocial barriers that decrease their occupational performance and quality of life (Nossum et al., 2017; Uzogara, 2017). Current evidence suggests a weight-inclusive approach to healthcare but there is still a significant amount of anti-fat bias that leads to learned helplessness, avoidance in participation of occupational roles, and avoidance in seeking primary healthcare services (Barclay & Forwell, 2018; Hunger et al., 2020). There is a lack of evidence on the contribution of occupation-based interventions for the obese population (Nielsen & Christensen, 2018). This may be due to the anti-fat attitudes that can be seen within occupational therapy (OT) students and professionals (Friedman & VanPuymbrouck, 2019). A look into a systematic review of programs involving occupational therapists shows successful improvements in QoL, improvements in performance, satisfaction, and health promotion when working with children and elders, and within family therapy for obese children (Bagaglini et al., 2019). Yet another scoping review of OT interventions for overweight and obese adults found that most focused on weight reduction (Nielsen & Christensen, 2018). This may be a reason for the lack of OT contribution to this population since weight regain is so common (Hall & Kahan, 2018).

Learning Activity:

How can this problem statement paragraph be refined for greater clarity or more directly linked to the profession of occupational therapy?

Images for This Chapter

The capstone is like putting a puzzle together. At this point, you have picked the puzzle off the shelf. You have a population or problem to pursue (for example, employment for individuals with severe mental illness or ASD).

In this chapter, you will begin to pull out the edge pieces of the puzzle to get the frame of a narrowed problem that can be framed in the timing of the capstone project.

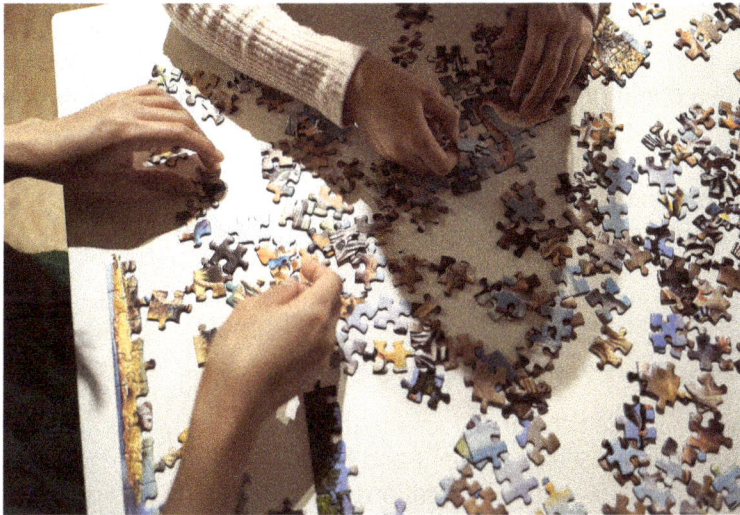

Figure 5.2 Completing a Puzzle

THE EVIDENCE-INFORMED PROBLEM – FINDING THE EDGES OF THE PUZZLE

Step 1: Find research articles that are relevant: Start by looking through academic databases, Google Scholar, or well-known journals. Look for articles written in the last few years that have something to do with your capstone project area of interest.

Step 2: Read the following: Abstract, discussion, and conclusion.

Step 3: Cut and paste or type in the information that answers the questions in the Literature Review Grid (see Worksheet 4.1).

Step 4: To find a current problem, look at column 4. What did the authors of the articles you read indicate should be done next to improve the population or problem being studied?

Step 5: Copy and paste the information from column 4 into a separate document. This will give you a clearer picture of what the authors think should happen in the future.

Step 6: Find patterns and common themes. Look for places where at least two authors suggest more services, further research, theory development, etc. are needed in the future. Having two authors who identify similar implications for the future indicates that this is a likely next step or gap to fill.

By following this process, you can find an evidence-informed problem for your capstone project, since the implications for the project can be defended by the current research articles.

EXAMPLE 1

See the Literature Review Grid in Chapter 4.

EXAMPLE 2: PROBLEM STATEMENT

Sentence 1: 'The problem is_____ which results in (OR which is a problem because) _____ (Citation 1, Citation 2) (Main idea sentence/topic sentence – summarize the main point of the paragraph).

Sentences 2–4: Supporting sentences – synthesize and support with citations information to increase the readers' depth of understanding with details about sentence 1. (Ensure the problem is clearly stated, links to the purpose, project, and profession. There must be a minimum of two current peer review articles supporting that this is a problem.)

Last sentence: Summarize the purpose of the paragraph and transition to the next paragraph or the next header.

Editing note: This section is generally 1–2 paragraphs.

FAQS

How Can I Find Relevant Literature Efficiently?

In the beginning, Google Scholar is your friend in this journey. Google Scholar has features that make an initial search efficient and broad (See Example 1). The ability to scan abstracts and learn about current publications quickly is a plus. The downside of Google Scholar is that there is an abundance of sources, and not all the sources are scholarly.

Using the features of Google Scholar, limit the articles by year of publication and scan the literature identified. Find your favorite 2–3 articles and look at the key terms that were used to link to those articles. After you have a better idea of key terms that are used surrounding an area of interest, take those key terms to use the databases available at your academic institution such as ProQuest or ERIC. The benefits of using your professional databases is library databases are categorized into an area of study, and there were professionals who organized and categorized the research articles. Use of the library databases usually means you will be able to open and read the entire article, or request it through the library services.

REFERENCES

American Occupational Therapy Association (2020). Occupational Therapy Practice Framework: Domain and Process – Fourth Edition. *American Journal of Occupational Therapy*, *74*(sup_2), 7412410010. https://doi.org/10.5014/ajot.2020.74S2001.

Ho, Y. R., Chen, B. Y., & Li, C. M. (2023). Thinking More Wisely: Using the Socratic Method to Develop Critical Thinking Skills Amongst Healthcare Students. *BMC Medical Education*, *23*(1), 173.

Huescar Hernandez, E., Moreno-Murcia, J. A., Cid, L., Monteiro, D., & Rodrigues, F. (2020). Passion or Perseverance? The Effect of Perceived Autonomy Support and Grit on Academic Performance in College Students. *International Journal of Environmental Research and Public Health*, *17*(6), 2143.

Schippers, M. C., Morisano, D., Locke, E. A., Scheepers, A. W., Latham, G. P., & de Jong, E. M. (2020). Writing About Personal Goals and Plans Regardless of Goal Type Boosts Academic Performance. *Contemporary Educational Psychology*, *60*, 101823.

Selvia, A. (2020). A Socratic Teaching Method to Foster Critical Thinking Skills among Nursing Students in Our Clinical Classroom Settings. *South Asian Research Journal of Nursing and Healthcare*, *2*(4), 1–11.

6

Finding a Mentor for a Capstone Research Project

> The capstone (the project and experience) is mentored by individuals with expertise in the area of interest (ACOTE, 2023). The mentor does not have to be an OT.
>
> The capstone experience takes place in a 'mentored practice setting' where mentorship is evident over the course of the experience.

WHAT IS A MENTOR?

The capstone project requires students to have at least one formal mentor with expertise in their area of interest to guide them through the capstone journey. There are many definitions of mentor; the one used in this workbook is: 'a person with expertise consistent with the student's area of interest' (ACOTE, 2023).

In a broad sense, a mentor is someone who helps a mentee learn about something in a more efficient way (Zachary & Fain, 2022).

FORMAL VS. INFORMAL MENTORING

Mentoring can involve formal or informal arrangements where a person who is more experienced (mentor) helps in the personal and/or professional development of a person (mentee) who is less experienced.

Formal mentoring is structured by those involved, and for the capstone, verified by the academic institution. An informal mentoring relationship is initiated at a personal level and lacks structure. Table 6.1 demonstrates the differences between the two types of mentoring.

CHARACTERISTICS OF EFFECTIVE MENTORS

- Excellent supervisory skills
- Ability to empower the student
- Connected to support of the student
- Have conflict management skills
- Communication skills (receptive, approachable, and clear)
- Can honor the student's need for autonomy
- Ability to identify available opportunities in organizational networks
- Creates time for the mentee
- Expertise in the area of student interest.

DEVELOPING A FORMAL MENTORING ARRANGEMENT

The structure of formal mentoring arrangements can occur in various ways. Here is a brief overview of some of the types that can be relevant to the capstone.

Table 6.1 Formal versus Informal Mentoring

Formal Mentoring	Informal Mentoring
The organization recognizes the allocated time and commitment	In most cases allocated time and commitment is not recognized and long-term planning can be a challenge
Mentoring relationships take a given period (for instance, 9 to 12 months)	Flexible and can adapt to upcoming events or goals. It may be long-term or occasional
The strategic pairing of mentors and protégés	Individual picking of mentors and mentees
Everyone with qualifications can access	The mentor or mentee must initiate. May take place naturally without being considered as such
Offers continuous support and guidance as a co-coordinator, as well as support for all who are involved	Often lacks support or training
There is an evaluation/review process	Lacks formal evaluation of effectiveness
Measurable objectives	Flexible goals with adaptable objectives
Linked to a strategic outcome	Personal objectives, but do not have to be strategically aligned
Facilitated and backed by the organization	Developed on their own and do not form part of a program that is structured

One-on-One Mentoring

One-on-one mentoring often involves relationships between two individuals where one has more experience in areas of interest that the other person needs to develop in. This model is often applied in the majority of formal mentoring arrangements.

Group Mentoring

This type of mentoring involves a group of students who take part in a mentoring relationship with one mentor. Although individual students may have individual learning outcomes, there is an identified expertise of the mentor to meet both a group objective and individual student objectives.

Team Mentoring

Team mentoring is a situation where a group of mentors work collaboratively to mentor an individual mentee or group of mentees. The members come together to present mutual learning outcomes and collaborate simultaneously with single or multiple mentors who take mentees through an intentional process to support their knowledge acquisition. The process of mentoring enables the team to learn from every member's knowledge and experience.

MENTORING BENEFITS

Various research findings have demonstrated desired outcomes for career satisfaction and success for both mentees and mentors (Keramidas et al., 2022). The benefits of mentoring vary from one student to another. Some of the most common benefits include:

Benefits for Mentees

- Enhancing self-awareness and professional confidence
- Tapping mentor's expertise and amassed knowledge
- Acquiring insight into the culture and norms of an institution and discovering the ways of operation, including rules that are 'unwritten'
- New insight into individual practices and behavior
- Finding a role model
- Increasing visibility and expanding networks
- Minimizing feelings of isolation
- Student-initiated mentorship improves many professional personality traits (Keramidas et al., 2022).

Benefits for Mentors

- Personal growth and satisfaction
- The opportunity to enhance leadership and communication skills
- Expanding their professional network
- The ability to explore new perspectives
- Developing a potential for a legacy or contribution in the profession.

THREE COMMON TYPES OF CAPSTONE MENTORS

Students will have a minimum of one formal mentor during the capstone. This means that before the experience begins, there will be documentation and verification of a mentor in relation to the student capstone. Students can have more than one formal mentor; for example, a subject matter expert to mentor the project, and a site mentor to provide mentorship at the practice setting.

1. Faculty Mentor

A faculty mentor is an experienced professor who guides, advises, and supports the student mentee through the development of the capstone project and experience (Allen et al., 2006; Almond et al., 2021). Students may develop professional relationships with many faculty members over the capstone development process. Faculty members may be formal or informal mentors.

Collaboration with faculty members is essential to the development of the capstone project and experience. Therefore, students are encouraged to reach out to faculty for guidance throughout the development process. Faculty will collaborate with students in planning, developing, and implementing. Some faculty will serve as informal mentors alongside the development process, while one faculty member may serve as the formal mentor. Similar to all mentor types, a faculty member serving as the formal mentor will be documented and verified for the individual student project and experience.

Pros and cons of a faculty mentor: Asking a faculty member you know from class to be a capstone mentor offers the advantage of familiarity. Potential downsides include faculty mentoring multiple students and their field of interest being different from their students'.

2. Subject Matter Expert (SME)

A subject matter expert (SME) is a person who has qualifications or experiences in a certain area or system that align with the student's area of interest. A SME's qualification can be verified from their education, training, or experience. The SME provides oversight and input to the development of the capstone.

Pros and cons of a SME: A SME brings current, specialized knowledge to the capstone. This knowledge and expertise can facilitate the capstone project and deepen the student's understanding of the topic. The SME can streamline the process by discussing the area of interest with depth and breadth. However, despite their expertise in a certain area, a SME may not be well-versed in every aspect of the student's area of interest. In addition, they may be unfamiliar with the academic program and capstone requirements, necessitating additional time to explain mentorship expectations.

3. Site Mentor

A site mentor is someone who has the role of a mentor and/or supervisor during the capstone experience. A site mentor frequently is an employee at a particular location who provides guidance and mentorship to students within that setting. This method, known as site-based mentoring, allows students to become fully immersed in the facility's operations.

Pros and cons of a site mentor: One of the most significant benefits of having a site mentor is the extensive opportunities it affords students. A site mentor can network the student into different aspects of the organization. This mentor type can open the door for a student to engage in diverse types of learning opportunities. However, a site mentor's perspectives and practices may focus on their facility. The focus on one facility may limit exposure to broader problems and practices.

A student can benefit from having multiple (formal or informal) mentors with diverse areas of expertise. An individual mentor can serve as a site mentor who guides practical experience, a subject matter expert who imparts specialized knowledge, and a faculty member who provides guidance on academic perspectives. It is not uncommon for a mentor to simultaneously embody multiple roles, reflecting the multifaceted qualities they possess. Seeking multiple mentors, in addition to the required formal mentor and site supervisor, can enhance the depth and breadth of the capstone project and experience.

WHAT ATTRIBUTES DO YOU BRING TO THE MENTORED EXPERIENCE? IN ADDITION TO MEETING YOUR NEED FOR AN EXPERIENCE, WHAT WILL YOU BE DOING FOR YOUR SITE/MENTOR WHILE YOU ARE THERE?

Mentoring is a two-way street. Meaning both the mentor and the mentee should benefit from a mentorship relationship. Apart from benefiting from the mentoring experience as a student, you need also to have something that you can offer to your mentor/site in the process.

Mentees/students are a source of feedback and fresh perspectives to mentors while enhancing their growth and leadership skills. Just like mentors, the attributes of mentees vary. Some important attributes the student should be prepared to demonstrate are:

- Be respectful of your mentor's resources and time
- Be ready to take risks, try new approaches, and be challenged
- Be dedicated to the mentoring process and focused on achieving objectives
- Be flexible in the opportunities the mentor might provide.

Use Worksheet 6.1 to reflect on and make a plan for mentorship.

FINDING A MENTOR FOR A CAPSTONE PROJECT AND EXPERIENCE

There are a variety of ways to find a mentor for a capstone project and experience.

1.   Read the Literature – Look at Authors

One of the ways you can find a mentor is by looking at the authors publishing on your area of interest. If you continue to read about your area of interest and notice there are one or two people publishing in your area of interest, consider reaching out to them. Take note of at least one aspect of the author's research that interests you and contact them to see if they would be willing to provide mentorship.

2.   Ask Faculty

Ask faculty who share expertise or experience in your area of interest. You don't have to have a prior relationship with faculty before approaching them for mentorship. Set up a time to discuss your area of interest with them.

3.   Google/Online Searches for People and Organizations that Align with Your Area of Interest

Use the World Wide Web. Google and search for organizations that align with your area of interest. Consider people or organizations that align with your area of interest at the individual, group, or population level. These options include people who work towards advocacy, program and policy development, or leadership. The mentor does not have to be providing one-to-one service to serve as a mentor. Consider mentors who work in the area of interest at different levels.

4.   Ask Peers

You can find a mentor by asking fellow students for ideas. Graduates or students who have completed a capstone in your area of interest may be able to serve as your mentor or connect you with their mentors. Classmates may have family and friends with access to an aspect of your area of interest. Often your peers can share contacts about mentors working in your field of interest.

HOW TO MAKE THE 'ASK'

As you approach a potential mentor, you should be ready for a 'yes', 'no' or 'let me think about it' response. Be ready to discuss what opportunity you are looking for from their mentorship.

Phone Call versus Email versus the Drive By

As a student, you have gone through all the processes, and you have identified a few potential mentors. Now you are ready to approach a potential mentor.

   After identifying a potential mentor, gather as much information as possible about him/her before reaching out. The most common way initial requests are made is via email. The content of the email will be different depending on the mentor type. Use Learning Activity 6.1 to draft an email to a potential mentor.

Learning Activity 6.1: Drafting an Email to a Potential Mentor

Table 6.2 Drafting an Email to a Potential Mentor

Faculty Mentor: Go to office hours, meet after class, or use some of the guidance for the other mentor types.

Subject Matter Expert (SME):
- Introduce yourself and explain how you came to know of the SME.
- State a clear purpose. Are you looking for the SME to be a project mentor, a site mentor, or both?
- Provide an overview of your project goals.
- Acknowledge their time and expertise.
- Provide options to exchange more information.
- Include your contact information.

Site Mentor:
- Introduce yourself and explain how you came to know about the potential mentor and site or facility.
- State a clear purpose. Are you looking for the mentor to mentor the project, the experience, or both?
- Provide an overview of your project and experiential goals.
- Acknowledge their time and expertise.
- Provide options to exchange more information.
- Include your contact information.

Request for Mentorship Regarding [Specific Topic]

Dear Dr./Mr./Ms. [Last name of potential mentor],

I hope that you are doing well. I am an OTD student at _____. I recently had the chance _____ [for example: to read your insightful article on (specific topic or title of article) or saw your company on the web] and was truly impressed by _____ [reason you would like them to be your mentor].

I'm reaching out to you because I am looking for a mentor to _____ [a brief description of your project or the specific challenge you're facing]. Given your extensive experience in this area, I believe your guidance could be invaluable.

Note: Include if you are asking for the mentor to be the mentor at the practice setting:

I am interested in learning more about _____ [area of interest] and I am hoping to have the opportunity to learn at _____ [name of site]. I would be looking for the opportunity to participate in activities [list specific departments or activities of interest] offered at [site].

I recognize that your time is valuable, and I would greatly value any advice or suggestions you could provide. Whether it's answering a few specific questions via email or scheduling a brief phone or video conversation, I'm flexible and would appreciate any format that best suits your needs.

If you are open to having a discussion about mentorship, please let me know when you are available to set up a potential call or meeting.

Option 1: [Time and Date]
Option 2: [Time and Date]
Option 3: [Time and Date]

Thank you so much for considering my request. I truly value the opportunity to learn from someone with your expertise in _____[specific field or topic]. Please feel free to contact me if you have any questions or require further information.

Warm regards,

[Your full name]

[Your contact information: Email, phone number]

Now the Email Is Sent

People are often very busy and do not respond immediately. Don't despair!

Follow-up phone calls are important after sending an email. Here is a general rule of thumb:

- Initial waiting period: After sending an initial email, wait 3–7 business days before sending a follow-up email. This gives the recipient time to review their emails, address any pressing matters, and respond.
- Send a follow-up email: It is courteous to send a follow-up email prior to making a phone call. This serves as a little reminder and provides the recipient with a second chance to respond via email. Wait an additional 3 to 5 business days following this second email.
- After the follow-up email and the waiting period, if there is still no response, it is appropriate to make a phone call. There may be a variety of reasons why they haven't gotten back to you, so be courteous and patient when calling. Initiate the call by introducing yourself, mentioning the email(s) you sent, and elaborating on the reason for your call.
- Recognize that individuals may be preoccupied or may have overlooked your email among others. Approach the phone call with understanding and adaptability. It is possible that the recipient intended to respond but was busy.
- Limit persistent calls: If after the phone call there is still no response or the response was vague, assess the situation. Extreme persistence can come across as pushy. Depending on the circumstances, you may choose to wait longer, try a different method of communication, such as 'driving by' to see the site or mentor in person, or move on.

It is essential in every circumstance that you consider the nature of your relationship with the recipient, the context of the email, and any external factors that may influence the response time.

Use Learning Activity 6.2 to track your communication with potential mentors.

YOU'VE GOT VERBAL ACCEPTANCE FROM A MENTOR – NOW WHAT?

Connect Mentor to the Academic Program

After securing a mentor, it is now time to connect your mentor to the academic program. Your academic program might have procedures to follow after receiving a verbal confirmation. You can use Learning Activity 6.3 to help you draft an email to a mentor who has verbally agreed to provide formal mentorship. Copy the doctoral coordinator in to the email.

Learning Activity 6.2: Tracking Communication with Potential Mentors

Table 6.3 Tracking Communication with Potential Mentors

Potential Mentor Name	Contact Information: Email, Phone Number, Website	Date of first contact	Date of second contact	Date of third contact	Comment

Learning Activity 6.3: Capstone Project Mentor Email Template

Dear (use appropriate title) Dr./Mr./Ms. [Last name of potential mentor],

My name is _____ [Student Name] and I am an entry-level occupational therapy student in the entry-level doctorate program at _____. I am writing to thank you for verbally agreeing to mentor my doctoral capstone project in the area of _____. [Provide a brief introduction] I began my entry-level doctorate program in _____ [e.g., Fall 2024) at _____. I first wanted to provide background information on me, so I am attaching my resume for your review. I am looking forward to developing and completing my capstone project and experience with your mentorship from [start date] to [end date].

I chose to do a doctoral project focusing on the area of _____ because my interest lies in serving _____ . My literature review has focused on the crossover between _____ and occupational therapy. I would appreciate any guidance you can provide on how to best prepare for this experience, such as readings I should complete or resources I should investigate.

I know _____[university] will be contacting you soon. I will be forwarding your contact information to them. How do you want to proceed? Do you want to communicate by email or talk by phone?

Thank you for the opportunity to work with you on my capstone project and _____ [experience.] I am looking forward to working with you.

Sincerely,
[Student Name]
[Telephone Number]
[Email]

Example Learning Activity 6.3: Tracking Communication with Potential Mentors

Table 6.4 Example of Tracking Communication with Potential Mentors

Potential Mentor Name	Contact Information: Email, Phone Number, Website	Date of first contact	Date of second contact	Date of third contact	Comment
Aiden Lundelius	A.Lundelius@example.com #123–456–6789	Date(X) – Email	Plan phone call on X+12	If I don't hear back by third date, I will stop by the site to get a point of contact.	
Barbara Martinez	B.Martinez@yahoo.com #123–456–6789	Date(X +5) – Email	X+5 Email	Plan phone call on X+12	If I don't hear back from option one, I will focus on this option.

After the confirmation you will likely need an individualized mentor agreement.

Purpose of a Mentor Agreement

The goal of a mentor agreement is to verify the expertise of the mentor aligns with the 'student's area of focus prior to the onset of the doctoral capstone experience' (ACOTE, 2023).

During the initial steps in developing a relationship with a formal mentor, a main objective is to develop an understanding of mutual goals and expectations. A mentoring agreement is created by both the student and mentor to ensure that both comprehend the relationship's expectations and parameters of accountability. A mentoring agreement enhances a sense of ownership of the mentoring relationship, and it is an important tool to highlight mutual expectations. Chapter 13 of this workbook is dedicated to writing objectives. The initial objective will go into the mentor agreement. It is understood that objectives will change and evolve over the duration of the capstone project or experience. Use the mentor agreement to outline initial targeted goals. Use Learning Activity 6.4 to draft a mentor agreement.

Learning Activity 6.4: Draft a Mentor Agreement

Note: The academic institution will have templates for mentor agreements. Each student should use the one developed by the institution. This is only a sample.

I (We) [Mentor name(s)]:

_____

Agree to the following:

1. I will serve as the Doctoral Capstone Mentor for [Student Name], as the mentor for the capstone experience known as the 'mentored practice setting' starting from [start date] to [end date].
   Optional: Additionally, I will serve as the mentor for the development of the capstone project.
2. I will provide advice and resources to the student as needed regarding the [identified area of expertise].
3. I will schedule and participate in mentoring meetings with my mentee at least once a [day, week, month] from [start date] to [end date] either face to face, virtually, by phone, or via another negotiated form of contact.
4. I will collaborate to establish goals prior to the onset of the capstone experience and provide feedback and guidance towards the student, meeting the agreed-upon objectives.
5. I will communicate with the Doctoral Capstone Coordinator regarding any concerns or needs during the experience.
6. I will provide evidence of my expertise in the identified area (example: CV).

Student Signature _____   Date_____

Capstone Mentor Signature _____   Date _____

Doctoral Coordinator Signature _____   Date_____

DOCUMENTATION TYPES FOR DIFFERENT TYPES OF CAPSTONE MENTORS

Table 6.5 Possible Documentation Types for Different Types of Capstone Mentors

Mentor Type	Possible Mentor Agreement type	Considerations
Faculty Mentor	There may not be a mentor agreement	How is the faculty mentor selected? What type of mentorship does the faculty mentor provide during the experience? Summative, or formative, other. How does the faculty mentor's expertise align with your area of interest? How often will you meet with the mentor? Daily, weekly, biweekly? What objectives will be mentored?
Subject Matter Expert (SME)	There will likely be a signed mentor agreement.	How is the SME selected? By the academic program, by the student, or is there a collaboration? What type of mentorship does the SME provide during the experience? How does the SME mentor's expertise align with your area of interest? How often will you meet with the mentor? What objectives will be mentored?
Site Mentor	There will likely be a signed mentor agreement.	How is the site mentor selected? By the academic program, by the student, or is there a collaboration? What type of mentorship does the site mentor provide during the experience? How does the mentor's expertise align with your area of interest? How often will you meet with the mentor? What objectives will be mentored?

FAQs ABOUT FINDING A MENTOR(S)

1. **Who can I choose to be my mentor?**
   Choose a person who can help you realize and achieve your goals. This can be anyone with more expertise in your area of interest.
2. **Am I allowed to have more than one mentor?**
   Yes, you can establish more than one mentoring relationship. However, you should be selective to ensure you only choose mentors who match your mentoring needs.
3. **Can I end a mentoring relationship if the mentor does not match my mentoring needs?**
   In some instances, you might realize that your mentor is not suitable for your needs. In such a case, you can be honest and discuss your decision with the mentor and Doctoral Capstone Coordinator. Thank your mentor for his/her time and start a search for another mentor.

4. **What should I do if I don't get a response from a potential mentor?**

In case you don't hear from the potential mentor, try to contact him/her through his/her contact details that you have. If he/she does not respond, discuss this with your DCC. If after some time the potential mentor is not responding, it is advisable to look for another mentor who matches your needs.

Worksheet 6.1: Mentor Selection Worksheet

Self-assessment:

1. What are my goals for this capstone?

   a. What mentorship would be helpful for the project?
   b. What mentorship would be helpful for the experience?
   c. As you plan, will you benefit from two formal mentors?

2. What specific expertise or guidance am I seeking in a mentor?

   a. Would you benefit more from guidance to work with a specific population?
   b. Would you benefit more from guidance to complete a specific type of project?

3. Research potential mentors:

   a. Within the guidelines of your academic institution, Google organizations that serve your population of interest.

List five organizations or professionals who align with your capstone topic:

1

2

3

4

5

4. Initial outreach:

   a. Write a clear email or draft conversation for initial outreach (Learning Activity 6.1).
   b. Include your capstone idea, why you are reaching out to them specifically, and what guidance you're seeking.
   c. You may not hear back from an email, be prepared to call or go to the setting in person (Learning Activity 6.2).

5. Prepare for a follow up response:

   a. List at least five questions to ask a potential mentor during your first meeting.
   b. For instance: What are your expectations from mentees? Have you guided a project similar to this before?

6. Feedback and iteration:

    a. After each potential mentor meeting, note what went well and what could be improved.

    b. Were there questions you wish you had asked? Add them for the next meeting.

7. Commitment level:

    a. How involved do you want your mentor to be (e.g., weekly check-ins, monthly meetings, feedback on specific deliverables)?

    b. Are they available and willing to commit to that level of involvement?

8. Backup options:

    a. If your first choice doesn't work out, who is your second choice? Third?

    b. Remember, it's crucial to have multiple options.

9. Finalize agreement:

    a. Once you have selected a mentor, draft a mentorship agreement or plan that outlines both parties' expectations, commitment levels, and communication preferences (Learning Activity 6.3).

This worksheet is meant to guide students through the process of identifying, reaching out to, and finalizing their mentorship relationship for their capstone. Adjustments can be made based on specific needs and institutional requirements.

REFERENCES

Accreditation Council for Occupational Therapy Education (ACOTE) (2023). 2023 Accreditation Council for Occupational Therapy Education (ACOTE®) Standards and Interpretive Guide. Retrieved from: https://acoteonline.org/accreditation-explained/standards/.

Allen, T. D., Lentz, E., & Eby, L. T. (2006). Mentorship Behaviors and Mentorship Quality Associated with Formal Mentoring Programs: Closing the Gap between Research and Practice. *Journal of Applied Psychology*, *91*(3), 567–578. https://doi.org/10.1037/0021-9010.91.3.567.

Almond, L., Parson, L., & Resor, J. (2021). Lessons from the Field: Graduate Student-faculty Mentoring In Family Science. *Family Relations*, *70*, 1600–1611. https://doi.org/10.1111/fare.12517.

Burgess, A., van Diggele C., & Mellis C. (2018). Mentorship in the Health Professions: A Review. *The Clinical Teacher*, 15(3), 197–202. https://doi.org/10.1111/tct.12756.

Johnson, W. B. (2007). Student-Faculty Mentorship Outcomes. In T. Allen & L. Eby (eds.), *The Blackwell Handbook of Mentoring: A Multiple Perspectives Approach* (pp. 189–210). Blackwell Publishing.

Keramidas, N. L., Queener, J. E., & Hartung, P. J. (2022). Forming Mentoring Relationships in Graduate Education: The Role of Personality. *Australian Journal of Career Development*, *31*(2), 118–129. https://doi.org/10.1177/10384162221107972.

Zachary, L. J., & Fain, L. Z. (2022). *The Mentor's Guide: Facilitating Effective Learning Relationships*. John Wiley & Sons.

7

Finding a Mentored Practice Setting

Finding the experiential site for a capstone can be like trying to find a four-leaf clover. The process involves searching for a location, and then finding a site that has the potential to give you as many opportunities as possible. Finding a site that gives you the opportunity to participate fully is like finding a pot of gold. What steps can you take to identify and schedule your capstone experiential site?

There are differences between academic institutions: Some programs will assign the experiential site. If this is the case, you can skip to the next chapter!

The goal of the capstone experience is to have a 'concentrated experience in the designated area of interest' (ACOTE, 2023). If you can explore sites to meet your learning goals, one of the hardest parts is planning. What opportunities do you want to have during your experience? You are about to graduate with a clinical doctorate, so you want to be practicing what you have learned from your classes and fieldwork. Although you will select a single project type, you can plan experiences that include all potential project types. Envision which skills you want to practice over the experiential time, such as leadership, advocacy, or administration skills, even if these are not your project type. The main consideration is that the capstone experience is not a third Level II fieldwork experience. Compare the goals of a Level II fieldwork experience to the goals of the capstone experience.

Table 7.1 Goals of Level II Fieldwork versus Capstone Experience

Level II Fieldwork *Fieldwork provides an in-depth experience in delivering occupational therapy services to clients with a focus on:*	***Capstone*** *The capstone project and experience provides in-depth exposure to:*
The application of purposeful and meaningful occupation and research	Clinical skills
Administration	Research skills
Management of occupational therapy services	Administration
Exposure to a variety of clients across the lifespan	Program development and evaluation advocacy
Exposure to a variety of settings	Education
	Leadership

Source: ACOTE, 2023

Use Worksheets 7.1 and 7.2 to consider the individualized learning objectives you have and the ones you would like to develop during the capstone experience. Start by looking at all the project types for inspiration.

As a rule of thumb, the Level II fieldwork requires students to evaluate and treat clients and groups at the individual and group levels. Level II fieldwork focuses on assessment, evaluation, intervention, discharge planning, and billing. This is distinctly different from the capstone experience that focuses on in-depth exposure to and practice of advanced skills in an area of your choosing.

Use the worksheets to consider individualized objectives you have or those that you would like to develop during the capstone experience. Start by looking at all the project types for inspiration. Next, look at resources available at your academic program. Where have other students gone for their capstone experiences? What partnership does your academic program have in the community? Do any of these sites serve the population or address problems related to your area of interest? Identify potential sites that will give you a chance to develop an in-depth understanding of the population or problem related to your area of interest. Look at the example of options for a mentored practice setting for a student with a goal of working with a neurological population in Table 7.2.

Table 7.2 Example of Potential Mentored Practice Settings for a Student Developing In-Depth Exposure (aka Site) to the Neurological Population of Individuals Who Have Had a Stroke

Exposure you would like to have during your capstone experience	*Location where this experience could be offered* *(Contact information)*	*Would this be full time, part time, or a field study (only a few hours or days)? Circle your goal* *This is a plan – at the end, there needs to be 14 weeks and 560 hours.*
1. Clinical practice skills	*The Mayo Clinic* provides extensive stroke rehabilitation programs, including physical, occupational, and speech therapy, as well as psychiatric counseling and family support for patients. (https://www.mayoclinic.org/) *The Kessler Institute for Rehabilitation* is a premier rehabilitation facility that provides specialist stroke rehabilitation programs, such as intensive inpatient care and outpatient therapy services. (https://www.kessler-rehab.com/) *Spaulding Rehabilitation Hospital* is a Harvard-affiliated facility that provides comprehensive stroke rehabilitation programs, including inpatient and outpatient care, as well as patient and family support and education (https://spauldingrehab.org/).	Develop individual goals that align with the capstone experience. Be sure to differentiate your goals from fieldwork experience. full time (14 weeks/560 hours) part time (16 weeks/35 hours per week) = full time at one location OR part time (14 weeks/20 hours per week at one location and then 14 weeks/20 hours per week at another location – part time at 2 locations field study (only a few hours or days)

Table 7.2 (Continued)

Exposure you would like to have during your capstone experience	Location where this experience could be offered (Contact information)	Would this be full time, part time, or a field study (only a few hours or days)? Circle your goal This is a plan – at the end, there needs to be 14 weeks and 560 hours.
2. Research skills	*The National Institute of Neurological Disorders and Stroke (NINDS)* is a federal agency that funds study into neurological conditions, such as strokes. For students, they provide research opportunities and training courses. (https://www.ninds.nih.gov/) *The American Heart Association (AHA)* supports research into cardiovascular disorders, including stroke. For college students interested in studying strokes, they provide grants and fellowships for research. (https://www.heart.org/) *The American Stroke Association (ASA)* is a branch of the American Heart Association that specializes in stroke care. Students interested in studying stroke research can apply for opportunities. (https://www.stroke.org/)	Pick one: full time (14 weeks/560 hours) part time (16 weeks/35 hours per week) = full time at one location OR part time (14 weeks 20 hours per week at one location and then 14 weeks 20 hours per week at another location – part time at 2 locations field study (only a few hours or days)
3. Administration	*The National Stroke Association (NSA)* is a nonprofit group that offers services and education about strokes. Through internships and volunteer work, they give students the chance to hone their managerial and leadership abilities. (https://rarediseases.org/organizations/national-stroke-association/) *The American College of Healthcare Executives (ACHE)*. For students interested in hospital administration and leadership, they provide resources and opportunities, such as internships and mentorship programs. (https://www.ache.org/)	Pick one: full time (14 weeks/560 hours) part time (16 weeks/35 hours per week) = full time at one location OR part time (14 weeks 20 hours per week at one location and then 14 weeks 20 hours per week at another location – part time at 2 locations field study (only a few hours or days).
4. Leadership	*Healthcare Financial Management Association (HFMA)* is for healthcare financial management professionals and offers mentorship programs, leadership development opportunities, and educational resources. (https://www.hfma.org/) *Healthcare Information and Management Systems Society (HIMSS)* is an organization for healthcare information and technology professionals that offers mentorship programs, leadership development opportunities, and educational resources. (https://www.himss.org/who-we-are)	Pick one: full time (14 weeks/560 hours) part time (16 weeks/35 hours per week) = full time at one location OR part time (14 weeks 20 hours per week at one location and then 14 weeks 20 hours per week at another location – part time at 2 locations field study (only a few hours or days)

(Continued)

Table 7.2 (Continued)

Exposure you would like to have during your capstone experience	Location where this experience could be offered *(Contact information)*	Would this be full time, part time, or a field study (only a few hours or days)? Circle your goal This is a plan – at the end, there needs to be 14 weeks and 560 hours.
5. Program and policy development	Local community organizations that serve individuals who have experienced strokes that would allow a student to run a program and give feedback on strategies to develop institutional policies and procedures for sustainability of the program. Day treatment centers that would allow a student to run a program and give feedback on strategies to develop institutional policies and procedures for sustainability of the program. Independent or assisted living facilities that would allow a student to run a program and give feedback on strategies to develop institutional policies and procedures for sustainability of the program.	Pick one per site: full time (14 weeks/560 hours) part time (16 weeks/35 hours per week) = full time at one location OR part time (14 weeks 20 hours per week at one location and then 14 weeks 20 hours per week at one location – part time at 2 locations field study (only a few hours or days)
6. Advocacy	*Brain Aneurysm Foundation (BAF)* is a global organization that focuses on education, advocacy, and research. There are opportunities for advocacy, particiaption in grants, and research. (https://www.bafound.org/) *The American Stroke Association (ASA)* is a branch of the American Heart Association that specializes in stroke care. Internships and volunteer jobs give students the chance to get active in advocacy for people who have had strokes (https://www.stroke.org/en/). *National Aphasia Association*: focuses on public awareness, and research to improve the lives of people with aphasia. There are opportunities for research, education, grants, and advocacy. (https://www.aphasia.org/)	Pick one: full time (14 weeks/560 hours) part time (16 weeks/35 hours per week) = full time at one location OR part time (14 weeks 20 hours per week at one location and then 14 weeks 20 hours per week at another location – part time at 2 locations field study (only a few hours or days)
7. Education	Work with the National Stroke Association on their 'The Comeback: Stories of Stroke Recovery', series. This podcast features interviews with stroke survivors, caregivers, and healthcare professionals who share their experiences and insights on stroke recovery.	Pick one: full time (14 weeks/560 hours) part time (16 weeks/35 hours per week) = full time at one location

Table 7.2 (Continued)

Exposure you would like to have during your capstone experience	Location where this experience could be offered (Contact information)	Would this be full time, part time, or a field study (only a few hours or days)? Circle your goal This is a plan – at the end, there needs to be 14 weeks and 560 hours.
		OR part time (14 weeks 20 hours per week at one location and then 14 weeks 20 hours per week at another location – part time at 2 locations field study (only a few hours or days)
8. Theory development	Work with a recognized occupational therapist developing a theory to further the development and application of a theory. Attend conferences and seminars on occupational therapy theory development. Students could take part in existing research studies that advance the theory of occupational therapy. This may entail participating in the design and execution of research investigations, evaluating data, and interpreting findings.	Pick one per site: full time (14 weeks/560 hours) part time (16 weeks/35 hours per week) = full time at one location OR part time (14 weeks 20 hours per week at one location and then 14 weeks 20 hours per week at another location – part time at 2 locations field study (only a few hours or days)

WHAT ARE YOUR UNIVERSITY'S REQUIREMENTS?

There are two primary ways a student secures their mentored practice setting (aka experiential site where they can develop an in-depth understanding of the population/problem or project type). A university can have the student identify sites or the university can assign sites, or there may be a collaborative approach.

Top Reasons It Is Beneficial to Find Your Own Capstone Experience Site (with Assistance from the Doctoral Coordinator or Mentor)

Securing your own capstone experience site allows you to take an active role in your education, ensuring the learning experience meets your individualized goals.

The student gains several advantages by securing their own capstone experience site:

1. Customized learning experience: By choosing their own experience site, students can choose an environment that best matches their interests and goals. This enables them to personalize their learning experience and concentrate on topics that are most relevant to their capstone and future career.

2. Students are encouraged to take a more self-directed approach to their learning by taking responsibility for securing their own capstone experience site. This promotes independence and aids in the development of skills required for lifelong learning.

3. Opportunities for networking: Choosing their own capstone experience site allows students to connect with professionals in their field. This can result in valuable networking opportunities and may open doors to future career opportunities.

4. Students are more likely to be motivated and engaged in their learning when they take an active role in their own education. This can result in improved outcomes and a more enjoyable educational experience.

5. Develops problem-solving skills: When a student finds and gets their own internship, they have to deal with any problems that come up. This helps them develop problem-solving skills that they can use in their future careers.

6. Develops initiative: Getting an internship on your own shows that you have initiative and are taking charge of your own education and career development.

7. Self-confidence: Doing an internship on your own can help you feel good about yourself and proud of what you've achieved.

8. Improves communication skills: When a student looks for an internship on their own, they have to communicate well with possible internship sites. This helps them improve their communication skills.

9. Increases independence: Getting an internship without help shows how independent a student is and how well they can manage their own education and career development.

10. Develops networking skills: When a student finds an internship on their own, they can meet professionals in their field and build relationships with them. This can lead to future job opportunities.

11. Improves adaptability: When a student finds and gets an internship on their own, they have to adjust to new places and situations. This makes them more adaptable and flexible.

12. Encourages a growth mindset: Students who learn on their own and set their own goals are more likely to have a growth mindset, which is important for success in school and in the workplace.

Top Reasons It Is Beneficial for a Student to be Assigned Their Capstone Experience Site (with Assistance from the Doctoral Coordinator or Mentor)

When a university assigns a capstone experience site, the student needs to take the initiative to make their capstone project unique. This can be done through student-centered learning, in which the student is at the center of the learning process and takes an active role in it. By getting involved in their capstone project, students can make it relevant to their own interests and career goals.

This can be done by having each student set their own goals and doing activities that focus on them. The student must be able to learn on their own and be responsible for their own education and career growth. By setting individual project and experiential goals, the student can improve their critical thinking, problem-solving, time management, and communication skills. This personalized, student-centered learning can help students develop a growth mindset and further their careers.

Here are some top reasons it is beneficial to be assigned a capstone experience site:

1. Personalize the experience: Knowing the site in advance, a student can make their internship experience meaningful and relevant to their own interests and career goals by setting individual goals within the assigned site. These goals may be focused on the project type versus the population.

2. Continuity of the project: Building an individual project at an existing site allows for student projects to develop over the years.

3. Consistency and familiarity: Since there is already a relationship between the academic institution and the capstone site, this provides a level of consistency and familiarity that can facilitate more effective communication and collaboration.

4. Sustainability: With an established system and relationship, there is a greater possibility that the project will be sustainable over the long term.

5. Benchmarks: As a result of the established relationship between the academic institution and the site, quality benchmarks are frequently in place, ensuring that the capstone experience meets a high standard.

6. Availability of resources: The established relationship can facilitate access to resources, such as equipment or expert consultation, that would otherwise be difficult to obtain.

7. Reduced onboarding time: Familiarity between the institution and the site could expedite the onboarding process, allowing students to begin working on their projects sooner.

8. Streamlined feedback loop: The pre-existing relationship facilitates a more effective feedback process, which can be crucial given the iterative nature of capstone projects.

9. Learning objectives: Since the academic institution is familiar with the capstone site, the learning objectives can be more closely aligned with the site's unique opportunities and challenges.

HOW TO MAKE THE 'ASK'

As you approach a potential facility or site/mentored practice setting, you should be ready for a 'yes', 'no', or 'let me think about it' response. Be ready to discuss what opportunities you are looking for from an experience at an organization.

Phone Call versus Email versus the Drive By

After identifying a potential facility or site/mentored practice setting, gather as much information as possible about the organization before reaching out. The most common way initial requests are made is via email. Use Learning Activity 7.1 to draft an email to introduce yourself. However, organizations are busy and if a target organization doesn't respond to an email, make a phone call. If there is no response then 'drive by' by walking in to the organization's offices or facility and introducing yourself, if this is possible.

To prepare for a phone call, identify two or three services at the organization that you would be interested in participating in. Describe how you would support the organization in the context of the service. To prepare for the drive by, in addition to preparing a one-minute speech about the services you would like to participate in, ensure you are dressed appropriately.

Learning Activity 7.1: Drafting an Email to a Potential Mentored Practice Setting

- Introduce yourself and how you came to know the organization.
- State a clear purpose. What area, program, department, etc., are you interested in pursuing?
- Provide an overview of your experiential goals for that organization.
- Acknowledge their time and expertise.
- Provide options to exchange more information.
- Include your contact information.

Request for Capstone Experience (Use Words Such as Internship for Non-OT Locations): [Specific Topic]

Dear Dr./Mr./Ms. [Last Name of Potential Mentor],

I hope that you are doing well. I am an OTD student at _____. I am reaching out to express my interest in pursuing an internship at _____ [organization] in _____ [department].

I'm reaching out to you because my chosen area of interest for my capstone is _____ [area of interest] and your organization _____ [what organization does that aligns with area of interest]. I am interested in learning more about how your organization serves _____ [the population] both for individuals, and in the community. I would be looking for the opportunity to participate in activities _____ [list specific departments or activities of interest] offered at _____ [site].

I recognize that your time is valuable, and I would greatly value any advice or suggestions you could provide. Whether it's answering a few specific questions via email or scheduling a brief phone or video conversation, I'm flexible and would appreciate any format that best suits your needs.

If you are open to having a discussion about an internship, please let me know when you are available to set up a potential call or meeting.

Option 1: [Time and Date]
Option 2: [Time and Date]
Option 3: [Time and Date]

Thank you so much for considering my request. I truly value the opportunity to learn from someone with your expertise in _____ [specific field or topic]. Please feel free to contact me if you have any questions or require further information.

Learning Activity 7.2: Tracking Communication with Potential Mentored Practice Settings/Sites

Table 7.3 Tracking Communication with Potential Mentored Practice Settings/Sites

Potential Facility	Contact Information: Email, Phone Number, Website	Date of First Contact	Date of Second Contact	Date of Third Contact	Comment

_____

_____

_____

_____

_____

_____

Learning Activity 7.2 Example: Tracking Communication with Potential Mentored Practice Settings/Sites

Table 7.4 Example of Tracking Communication with Potential Mentored Practice Settings/Sites

Potential Facility	Contact Information: Email, Phone Number, Website	Date of First Contact	Date of Second Contact	Date of Third Contact	Comment
Parkinson's center at any town	Parkinson Center.com Name	Date(X) – Email	X+5 – Email	Plan phone call on X+12	If I don't hear back by third date, I will stop by the site.
Parkinson's Foundation	Parkinson ofundation. com Name	Date(X +5) – Email	X+5 – Email	Plan phone call on X+12	If I don't hear back from option one, I will focus on this option.

Next look at resources available at your academic program. Where have other students gone for their capstone experience? What partnership does your academic program have in the community? Do any of these sites serve the population or address problems related to your area of interest? Identify potential sites that will give you a chance to develop an in-depth understanding of the population or problem that is your area of interest.

Worksheet 7.1: Student Self-Evaluation

Searching for a Mentored Practice Setting

Find your area of interest, i.e., what part of occupational therapy you are most interested in and where you would like to learn more. This could mean working with a certain group of people, in a certain type of practice, or on a certain kind of project.

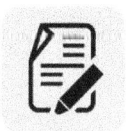

List your top three areas of interest:

1

2

3

What project type or types would you like to pursue? If you are doing an advocacy-type project, look at advocacy-type organizations; if you are doing a leadership-type project, look at organizations that align with the type of leadership skills you want to experience.

From your areas of interest what project type might you pursue?

1

2

3

Look into possible settings. Look into places that fit with your area of interest and the project type. Talk to OT professionals in the area, search online, or look at the websites of national, state, and local organizations.

From your areas of interest and project type, identify three potential sites where you could envision participating for 14 weeks and 560 hours.

1

2

3

OPTIONAL: You get to create an individual capstone experience. If there is more than one learning opportunity you would like to pursue, how many hours would you spend at different locations? You could pick two locations or incorporate an additional experience for short periods of time. If you go to alternate locations, this is considered 'off-site from the mentored practice setting.'

If you would like more experiential learning and planned for two mentored practice settings, what are potential sites?

1

2

3

Worksheet 7.2: Finding Potential Experiential Sites

Identify your population or problem of interest: _____
During your 14-week capstone experience, which of the following would you like to have exposure to? (Circle all that apply)

Clinical practice skills   Administration
Research skills   Program and policy development
Leadership   Advocacy
Education   Theory development

Table 7.5 Exposure

Exposure to the Following	*Ranked Priority (If the project type must be accomplished at the site, then this should be ranked #1)*	*Comments*

Prioritize the top types of experiences/exposures you would like to create for yourself. Search for organizations that could provide that experience. Write their contact information down, and when you are ready, start contacting the organizations in that order.

NOTE: The capstone experience is designed to provide students with opportunities to integrate and apply the knowledge and skills they have gained throughout their program. This is different from the Level II experience which focuses on developing and refining clinical practice skills through evaluation, treatment, and discharge of patients. The capstone experience cannot be developed as another Level II FW (fieldwork) experience.

Table 7.6 Prioritizing Exposure

Exposure you would like to have during your capstone experience	*Location where this experience could be offered (Contact information)*	*Would this be full time, part time, or a field study (only a few hours or days)*
1		
2		
3		
4		
5		

Worksheet 7.2 Example: Finding Potential Experiential Sites

Identify your population or problem of interest: **Reintegration Programs for Formerly Incarcerated Women**

During your 14-week capstone experience, which of the following would you like to have exposure to? (Circle all that apply)

Clinical practice skills   Administration
Research skills   **Program and policy development**
Leadership   Advocacy
Education   Theory development

Table 7.7 Example of Exposure

Exposure to the Following	Ranked Priority	Comments
Clinical Practice Skills	4	I would like to provide OT services using COPM and Occupational Profile to improve health and wellness at the individual or group level.
Research Skills	1	I would like this to be the capstone project type. I would like to explore how OTs work with individuals who are incarcerated, or formerly incarcerated. I don't know if the project will be qualitative or quantitative. I could collect data through virtual OT sites or focus groups. The research does not need to be done at the site.
Advocacy	3	I would like to spend time with an organization that works with individuals who are or were incarcerated.
Administration	5	If I am able, I would like to work with administration to learn the administration challenges.

Prioritize the top types of experiences/exposures you would like to create for yourself. Search for organizations that could provide that experience. Write their contact information down, and when you are ready, start contacting your mentor in that order.

Table 7.8 Example of Prioritizing Exposure

Exposure you would like to have during your capstone experience	Location where this experience could be offered (Contact information)	Would this be full time, part time, or a field study (only a few hours or days)?
1. Research Skills	Virtual	Part time, a few hours a few times over the experience
2. Program and Policy Development	Halfway house Prison Friends of Returning Citizens Community Bridges Fact Team The Last Mile Local church which has prison services	Full time, with flexible hours

3. Advocacy	Friends of Returning Citizens Community Bridges Fact Team The Last Mile	Full time, with flexible hours
4. Clinical Practice Skills	Halfway house Prison Friends of Returning Citizens Community Bridges Fact Team The Last Mile Local Church who has prison services	Full time, with flexible hours
5. Administration	Friends of Returning Citizens Community Bridges Fact Team The Last Mile Local church which has prison services	Part time, with flexible hours

NOTE: The capstone experience cannot be developed as another Level II FW experience.

REFERENCES

Accreditation Council for Occupational Therapy Education (ACOTE) (2023). 2023 Accreditation Council for Occupational Therapy Education (ACOTE®) Standards and Interpretive Guide. Retrieved from: https://acoteonline.org/accreditation-explained/standards/.

American Occupational Therapy Association (2020). Occupational Therapy Practice Framework: Domain and Process – Fourth Edition. *American Journal of Occupational Therapy*, *74*(sup_2), 7412410010. https://doi.org/10.5014/ajot.2020.74S2001.

Huescar Hernandez, E., Moreno-Murcia, J. A., Cid, L., Monteiro, D., & Rodrigues, F. (2020). Passion or Perseverance? The Effect of Perceived Autonomy Support and Grit on Academic Performance in College Students. *International Journal of Environmental Research and Public Health*, *17*(6), 2143.

Morris, T. H. (2020). Experiential Learning – A Systematic Review and Revision of Kolb's Model. *Interactive Learning Environments*, *28*(8), 1064–1077.

van Lent, M., & Souverijn, M. (2020). Goal Setting and Raising The Bar: A Field Experiment. *Journal of Behavioral and Experimental Economics*, *87*, 101570.

8

From Thoughts to Words: Starting Your Capstone Write-Up

WRITING YOUR PROJECT

When you are ready to begin writing or typing your project, this chapter provides guidelines to facilitate the writing process. This includes common expectations from academic institutions and publishers, obstacles to writing, and guidelines to develop a plan to draft and edit your work with reduced stress. There will be different expectations at different academic institutions. This workbook provides guidance towards widely recognized categories seen in doctoral writing. For your consideration, Chapters 10–12 and 15–16 start with a 'menu' of commonly seen categories.

COMMON EXPECTATIONS

Traditionally, doctoral education includes writing a dissertation, which typically consists of five chapters. This facilitates the student's systematic approach to societal issues. While this extensive process takes three to five years it is more in-depth than what is expected of an entry-level OTD. In the entry-level or clinical doctorate, there is a variety of methods to meet expectations. There are academic programs that follow the formatting seen in traditional doctoral education, but the submission might be seen in individual assignments or portfolio rather than in development of chapters. By understanding the objectives of each section, you can reduce stress and streamline the editing process for each category.

Let's briefly describe the goals of each 'chapter.' Note: Academic programs may have some of these categories or may have additional writing requirements. You may also see these categories broken down into smaller sections within coursework.

Getting Started: The Background Often Synonymous with Chapter 1

> **Common Content for the Background Section**
>
> 1) Explaining the context of an issue, 2) Define the problem, 3) Define the purpose, 4) State the significance and/or rationale, and 5) Give a definitions of terms.

Chapter 1 is the chapter where you begin to identify supporting information towards identification of a problem and how the problem is relevant to occupational therapy. At the conclusion of Chapter 1, an outside reader should have a basic understanding of the context surrounding the problem, the specific problem being addressed by the capstone project, and the purpose of the project. The student should be comfortable describing the problem with support from current literature and be open to feedback when an area of the project doesn't make sense.

The Literature Review Often Synonymous with Chapter 2

> ### Common Content for the Literature Review Section
>
> 1) A synthesis of current literature about the population or problem of interest; 2) A synthesis of current literature about the current services and professionals addressing the population or problem of interest; 3) A synthesis of current literature about the gaps between the services being provided and the current problem; 4) The role of OT in addressing this gap or current problem; 5) A model, framework, or theory to frame the capstone project.

Chapter 2 is the chapter where current literature is summarized. Each section or APA header or theme for Chapter 2 should summarize a section of the literature on the topic of interest. This section is generally considered the most challenging chapter to write. It is likely that this chapter is the hardest since it is the chapter where the most learning occurs. A student must read sufficient current literature to understand the topic of interest, and then synthesize the literature so other people can also understand the problem. This chapter is also challenging because the writing must strictly represent findings from the literature and exclude personal opinions. Focusing only on synthesizing literature minimizes personal bias and provides a comprehensive understanding of the issue.

The Project Plan or Methodology Often Synonymous with Chapter 3

Chapter 3 is the chapter where a plan is developed of how the student is going to address the problem identified in Chapter 1 and in alignment with the supporting literature review in Chapter 2. The plan must have enough specificity that a review of the project can be understood by all involved in the project. The OTD is not a process where 'winging it' will suffice. A need must be described and supported by the evidence, in this case the literature. The need will be addressed by a project that must evidence a strategy that would support the profession of occupational therapy. An outside reviewer should be able to see how the project would be a project completed by an occupational therapist, versus a social worker or a psychologist. The student should be ready to receive feedback on ways to make the project as rigorous as possible within the time frame. Given there are eight categories of projects, the written requirements vary. Refer to Table 8.1 to observe the differences and similarities between written requirement for various types of projects.

Table 8.1 Common Content for the Project Plan/Methodology Section

Program and Policy Development-Type Projects	*Research Process-Type Projects*	*Advocacy-Type Projects*
Description of planned program and policy project	Description of planned research project	Description of planned advocacy project
Needs assessment (i.e., logic model)	Needs assessment (i.e., theory of change)	Needs assessment (i.e., logic model)
Description of setting (or site)	Research questions and hypotheses	Description of stakeholders
Plans for recruitment	Research design	Description of setting (or site)
Description of planned participants		Plans for recruitment and involvement of relevant stakeholders

(Continued)

Table 8.1 (Continued)

Program and Policy Development-Type Projects	Research Process-Type Projects	Advocacy-Type Projects
Description of measures for program evaluation plan	Description of planned participants	Description of planned stakeholders
Development and implementation plan	Plans for recruitment	Description of tracking measures to evaluate progress plan
Data analysis/evaluation process	Data collection method or instrumentation	Development and implementation plan
Plan to draft policy for sustainable program provision.	Data collection and storage	Data analysis/evaluation process
Plan for dissemination	Data analysis plan	Plan for sustainability and dissemination
	Plan for sustainability and dissemination	

After completing Chapter 3, which outlines the project plan and Chapter 4, which describes the outcome of your plan, the capstone experience will also be complete!

The Outcome, the Results, the Findings Often Synonymous with Chapter 4

Chapter 4 is written after the project is complete. This chapter marks a pivotal moment in your capstone journey, detailing the results or outcomes of your project. This section organizes and presents your outcomes, aligning them with the plans you described in Chapter 3. By clearly outlining your objectives and outcomes, you offer readers – including mentors, peers, and faculty – a clear understanding of your achievements. Chapter 4 is a comparison between your initial plans (Chapter 3), their actual execution, and your findings. If an objective wasn't met, it's alright. Write the objective as you planned it in Chapter 3 and describe what went well, and what the barrier was to meet the objective. This way future students and practitioners interested in your topic can strategize more effectively for their projects. Essentially, this chapter provides a factual account of what was and wasn't achieved based on Chapter 3's intentions. Refrain from incorporating opinions here. In summary, Chapter 4 traces the journey from objectives to outcomes, bridging your project plan to what actually happened. Given there are eight categories of projects, the written requirements vary. Refer to Table 8.1 to observe the differences and similarities between written requirements for various types of projects.

Triumphs and Takeaways: The Heart of Your OTD Capstone: Future Implications, Implications for the Future, or Summary of Findings Often synonymous with Chapter 5

Chapter 5 of a capstone project includes several common categories of information to provide a comprehensive and clear summary of the research and its broader impact. You will create a 'Summary of Findings' section that summarizes your most important findings. This is different than Chapter 4 since this reports on the data. Chapter 5 is where you get to say what was most important about your findings. This is the only place in the writing of the capstone where you have freedom to give your opinion regarding your current understanding about your area of interest. Based on your project, what are the implications for your project on the population, organization,

Table 8.2 Common Content for the Outcome/Results/Findings Section

Program and Policy Development-Type Projects	Research Process-Type Projects	Advocacy-Type Projects
Description of completed program and policy project	Description of completed research project	Description of advocacy project
Description of setting (or site) used	Research questions and hypotheses	Description of stakeholders
Describe how recruitment was completed	Research design	Description of setting (or site)
Aggregate description of participants	Description of participants	Plans for recruitment and involvement of relevant stakeholders
Aggregate description of measures from the program evaluation	Plans for recruitment	Description of stakeholders
Describe implementation of program and policy	Data collection method or instrumentation	Description of tracking measures to evaluate progress plan
Explain data analysis and evaluation process	Data collection and storage	Development and implementation plan
Describe status of the draft policy for sustainable program provision	Data analysis plan	Data analysis/evaluation process
	Plan for sustainability and dissemination	Plan for sustainability and dissemination

or society? What are practical, real-world applications of your project? A common category is 'Recommendations for the Future' where you get to say where you think future students or practitioners should focus their energy on to make progress within your area of interest. Your recommendations provide a road map for future projects and contribute to the continuous advancement of scholarly, evidence-based understanding and investigation.

HOW TO PLAN AND ORGANIZE LITERATURE TO MAKE THE WRITING EASIER

Once you are in graduate school there is an expectation that you can communicate effectively by writing. If you don't feel writing is your strong point, seek out resources from your academic program. There are also editing services that you can pay for such as Upwork, Scribbr or PaperTrue. These services will assist with formatting and editing but are only useful once you have a strong draft explaining and supporting your project.

Sedita (2023), describes The Process Writing Routine, with the first letter of each word standing for Think, Plan, Write, Revise. The division of time spent in each stage is 40% thinking and planning, 25% writing, and 35% revising. In most academic curricula, the thinking and planning process for the capstone project and experience extends over several terms. Since it takes time to develop an in-depth understanding of an issue, this might be your initial experience in conceptualizing, planning, and revising a substantial piece of work. Unlike other classroom assignments which tend to be confined to a single course within one term, this endeavor, and your comprehension of it, evolves over time. It's natural to feel frustrated if it seems lengthy to produce a well-articulated written piece. ***Anticipate this as a part of the process!*** The worksheets in this workbook will walk you through steps within the writing process. Start with Worksheet 8.1 to help improve your productivity and time management.

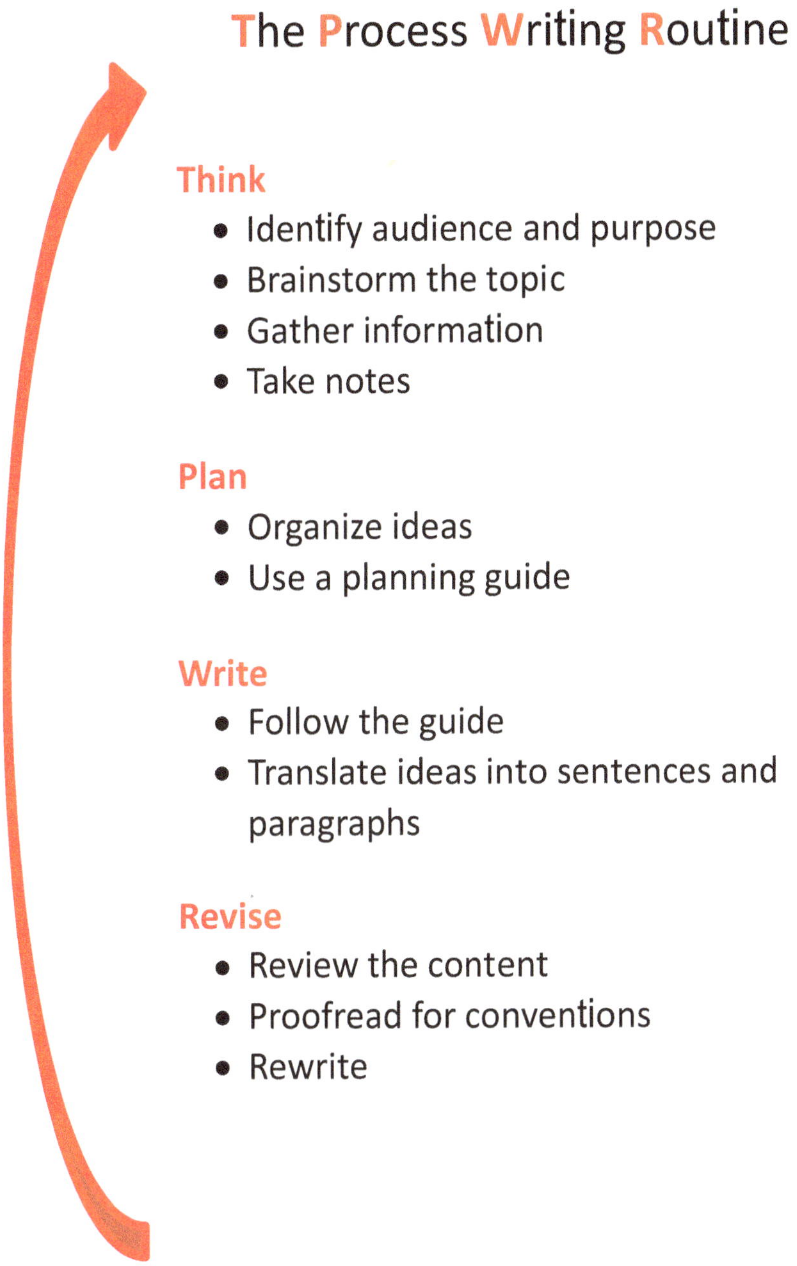

The Process Writing Routine

Think
- Identify audience and purpose
- Brainstorm the topic
- Gather information
- Take notes

Plan
- Organize ideas
- Use a planning guide

Write
- Follow the guide
- Translate ideas into sentences and paragraphs

Revise
- Review the content
- Proofread for conventions
- Rewrite

Figure 8.1 The Process Writing Routine
Source: https://keystoliteracy.com/blog/stages-of-the-writing-process/

Start by Thinking

Brainstorm what is the population, problem, or societal issue. *Read* the current literature related to your topic of interest. Extend your reading beyond just occupational therapy-specific literature. Familiarize yourself with the target population and explore the range of services and alternatives accessible to them. Seek to understand the prevailing challenges associated with your area of interest. The issue may be found at the level of an individual, group, organization, or population.

Track the literature you read. Utilize a literature grid (like the 'Literature Review Grid' in Chapter 4) or a management system such as Mendeley or Zotero. We recommend categorizing specific types of information starting from the beginning. We propose picking certain categories of information and tracking that information from each article. The advantage of consistently categorizing the same information from all sources is that you will need to reference different pieces of literature at various stages of writing. Having all of the literature organized in a single location simplifies the writing process.

Planning

Organize ideas. Develop categories of information that provide context to your area of interest. For clear organization, start by defining the goal of each section. For instance, the background section of Chapter 1 provides a concise overview of topics that will be explored in greater detail in Chapter 2. Next, outline the objective of every paragraph within that section. Finally, clarify the purpose of each sentence in the paragraph.

Use a planning guide (Worksheet 8.2) for each time you plan to write. This way you have a clear understanding of the goal of each section. Once you have a clear understanding of the goals of different sections of the writing, you can more effectively plan each paragraph or sentence.

Writing

Follow the directions from your academic institution. Use the templates and guidelines in Chapters 10, 11, and 12 provided in this workbook to plan and draft your thoughts into words.

Follow your plan from the planning guide. After you have a plan to write a section, focus only on that section.

Revising

As you keep reading the literature you will learn about your area of interest in more depth. After you learn more, you'll find the need to make revisions. You will also need to make revisions after receiving feedback from faculty. Remember, this type of writing is a continuous process, not a one-time effort. Plan for the revisions as part of the process.

OVERCOMING COMMON BARRIERS TO WRITING

There are known challenges to the writing process:

1. Lack of Clear Focus: Students start with a broad topic. At the beginning, it is challenging to narrow down a project to a specific direction. This is normal. As you keep reading, learning, writing, and editing, you will develop a clear, central problem to address for your capstone. Don't expect a clear focus from the beginning.
2. Procrastination and Time Management: Students may find it challenging to balance their time between reading and learning versus the writing and editing. We propose using assignment deadlines as guidelines for when to have drafts, and final drafts, ready for submission. We have observed that procrastination happens when students become immersed in reading and delay the actual writing. Finding a balance between the tasks requires time and practice. Utilize Worksheet 8.2 to establish your optimal writing times.

Remember, as you learn more, you will still be editing and can add in the new concepts in the editing process.

3. Information Overload: At the doctoral level, there is a wealth of literature and sources to explore. It's easy to become overwhelmed. As you read and learn more about an area of interest, there may not be a way to completely avoid this feeling. Over time, you will notice that the current literature surrounding your topic begins to sound repetitive. This is often termed as reaching a 'saturation point.' When you hit this milestone, first give yourself credit for reaching a saturation point as this means you've been putting in the work; it takes a lot of reading to reach this point. Also recognize that now you have a well-rounded understanding of your area of interest, which is a goal of doctoral capstone. Wills (2000) published a list of common personal barriers to writing and provided strategies to address them (see Table 8.3).

Table 8.3 Personal Barriers to Writing for Publication

Types of Personal Barrier	Strategies
Thoughts and Feelings	
Low motivation for writing; dearth of ideas for what to write	• Regularly read widely in areas of clinical research interests • Write about clinical issues of true personal interest • Don't assume findings or techniques are already known to others • Cultivate a sense of writing as an urgent, essential life priority • Partner with others and share writing tastes
Viewing self as an imposter; low confidence for publishing due to perceived lack of knowledge and skills	• Understand key gaps in knowledge for practice needing research • Read articles and books on writing for publication • Find a mentor and/or writing partners with complementary skills • Seek out classes, continuing education offerings, workshops • Remember that knowledge and skills develop only with practice
Fear of negative feedback or rejection	• Allow time for emotional reactions to feedback • Develop skills in not taking feedback personally • Seek support for feelings but don't dwell on catastrophic fears • Have objective colleagues provide input before submitting
Managing anxiety/frustration during writing	• View work *progress* as more important than work *pace* • Take frequent breaks and reward self for meeting due dates • Recognize perfectionism/unrealistic expectations as a pitfall • Balance writing with other activities that are restorative

LOOKING AHEAD

In conclusion, writing a capstone paper is a challenging but rewarding endeavor. Student writers will face challenges during the process. Personal growth will happen as you overcome each of the challenges. Remember that this is not a solitary journey; frequent feedback and interaction with peers and mentors are invaluable and will help you get through to graduation. Appreciate the learning process and the growth it brings. The reward will be in the culmination of a capstone project that makes a contribution to the profession of occupational therapy.

Worksheet 8.1: Capstone Writing Scheduling

Reflection Activity

Reason for activity: Professional writing is NOT easy. Don't underestimate the amount of thinking and time that are needed to develop a project worth pursuing (Graham, 2019; Kellogg, 2018).

Action items to consider:

Reflect on when you have had large assignments in the past. What was the time you found best to write?

What time of day has been most effective? _____
(Activity 1)

What days of the week will work best? _____
(Activity 2)

Can you write at home or do you work best by changing your environment? _____ Where do you write and focus best? Do you focus better in a cool or warm environment? Do you need silence or background noise? _____ (Activity 3)

What other tasks need to be cleared so you can focus on writing? _____ (Activity 4 – situational barriers)

What are strategies you can use to block the emotional challenges of life or anxiety about writing so the scheduled time can be used effectively? _____ (Activity 5 – personal barriers)

What supports do you have that help you write? For example: Do you write best with others or by yourself? _____

What barriers do you have to writing? For example, do you need to let your family know you will miss family dinner to open up the time to write effectively? _____

Plan to organize your literature in a way so that you don't need to organize it every time you sit down to write. For example, if you work at home, can you leave the paperwork out in the open so it is untouched until you sit back down to work? OR, if you go someplace to work, do you have tabbed notebooks so you can open up and start back up where you left off when the last session ended?

Use the activities below to plan when you will dedicate to the writing process:

Activity 1:

Select what time of the day you write best:

Table 8.4 Writing Times

	Check Off Your Best Writing Times	Plan Conditions that Must be Met to be Effective at this Time
4–6 AM		
6–8 AM		
8–10 AM		
10–12 PM		
12–2 PM		
2–4 PM		
4–6 PM		
6–8 PM		
8–10 PM		
10–12 PM/AM		

Activity 2:

Thinking of your current schedule, which days of the week will you be most available to work?

Fill in the times with tasks, such as attending class or sleep, that cannot be changed.

Table 8.5 Writing Schedule

	Sunday	Monday	Tuesday	Wednesday	Thursday	Friday	Saturday
4–6 AM							
6–8 AM							
8–10 AM							
10–12PM							
12–2PM							
2–4 PM							
4–6PM							
6–8PM							
8–10 PM							
10–12 PM/AM							

Worksheet 8.2: Planning Guide

Use this to plan each time you are sitting down to write.

Which section are you writing today? _____

How long is this section? _____

What is the purpose of this section? _____

When this section is complete, what is the main idea(s) the reader should know?

_____

_____

How many paragraphs do you think this section will be? _____
How many are you writing at one time? _____
What is the main idea of each paragraph?

Paragraph 1

Paragraph 2

Paragraph 3

Paragraph 4

Paragraph 5

If you need more than five paragraphs, consider if you have enough content for another section.

For each paragraph, what evidence or literature do you have to support what you are saying?

General rule of thumb:

Sentence 1: Main idea sentence

Sentence 2: Analysis sentence

Sentence 3: Evidence sentence (Use at least one citation)

Sentence 4: Evidence sentence (Use at least one citation)

Sentence 5: Conclusion and transition sentence

Revision

Consider self-revisions first. Read the section out loud so you can hear what you have written.

Consider a peer review. Ask a peer or family member to review your work. Stay receptive to their feedback, particularly about aspects they found clear or unclear. If you need to explain something to them verbally, consider writing down what you have said and putting that into the writing.

REFERENCES

Costa, A. D. (2021, August 16). Track How Much Time You Spent Editing a Word Document. *groovyPost*. Retrieved from: https://www.groovypost.com/howto/track-editing-time-microsoft-word-documents/.

Graham, S. (2019). Changing How Writing Is Taught. *Review of Research in Education, 43*(1), 277–303.

Kellogg, R. T. (ed.) (2018). Professional Writing Expertise. In *The Cambridge Handbook of Expertise and Expert Performance*. Cambridge University Press, p. 413

Purdue Writing Lab (n.d.). On Paragraphs // Purdue Writing Lab. Retrieved from: https://owl.purdue.edu/owl/general_writing/academic_writing/paragraphs_and_paragraphing/index.html.

Sedita, J. (2023). *The Writing Rope: A Framework for Explicit Writing Instruction in All Subjects*. Paul H. Brookes Publishing Co.

Wills, C. E. (2000, October). Strategies for Managing Barriers to the Writing Process. In *Nursing Forum*, *35*(4), 5–13.

Woolston, D. C., Robinson, P. A., & Kutzbach, G. (2020). *Effective Writing Strategies for Engineers and Scientists*. CRC Press.

9

Laying the Foundation

THE PROPOSAL, THE BACKGROUND, OR CHAPTER 1

The starting point for a capstone paper is for the student to provide a compelling case that the problem and project are worth pursuing. First, a case needs to be developed that explains the background or context of a population and the associated problem or need. Then, a clear statement of the problem and the purpose of the project needs to be explained with support from the evidence (literature). Finally, the purpose or project type will be outlined to help address or better understand this problem.

Each of these tasks might be called something different depending on your academic program. The case that supports your capstone project might be called a proposal, or each assignment might be collected individually, or not all of the sections may be required. For purposes of the workbook, we will refer to the 'compelling case' as Chapter 1, which aligns with common categories in doctoral writing.

Chapter 1 might include: a background, problem, purpose, rationale, significance, objectives, definitions, assumptions, delimitations, conclusion. They can be written together in one document or divided and written separately.

Menu

Use the menu of options below to understand what categories of information can be found when making a 'compelling case' to support your capstone project. Select options that align with the information you intend to include in making your compelling case.

Background: An overview of the context and previous research related to the area of interest. The goal of the background is to present information in a methodical way so the reader can understand your area of interest, the problem or need that exists, and what your project hopes to accomplish.

Conceptual or theoretical framework: The underlying principles or theories that guide and inform the project or identify frameworks being used in the literature.

Problem: A clear statement of the main issue or challenge the project seeks to address.

Purpose: A clear statement of how the main issue or challenge will be addressed. For the OTD this links to a project type.

Rationale: States the current need for the project by outlining potential contributions to problem, population, profession, and society. Answer the question, 'Why should anyone care about this project?'

Significance: Explains the intended effect(s) the project will have to address the problem. Describe the project's potential for positive change from the current situation for the population, phenomena, profession, or society.

Objectives: Specific goals the project aims to achieve.

DOI: 10.4324/9781003525868-10

Definitions: Clarifications of key terms and concepts used throughout the paper. If different authors use different definitions of key terms, identify the definition used in your paper.

Assumptions: Underlying beliefs or conditions considered true for the purpose of the project (Dusick, 2014).

Limitations: Assumptions or features the student cannot control. For example, the project must be completed in 14 weeks or less (Dusick, 2014).

Delimitations: Assumptions or features the student can control (Dusick, 2014).

Conclusion: A summary of all the main points that support pursuit of the individual capstone project.

OVERVIEW AND PREPARATION

Developing an occupational therapy capstone project proposal starts with reading literature as it allows students to get a depth and breadth understanding of their area of interest. Reading current literature is a step that can't be skipped. Developing an understanding about your area of interest, and learning what is currently being done, ensures you approach the problems with an aligned project type. For example, a systematic review of the literature on community mobility after spinal cord injury by Hitzig et al. (2021) found that there was a significant lack of research on the topic, which suggests that this is an area that would benefit from further study. If you didn't read literature, you wouldn't know where the current need is to improve the situation in your area of interest.

Reading Literature Is the First Step in Developing an Occupational Therapy Capstone Project

The Process is Cyclical

Step 1: To build a strong case for your project, you must read literature to understand the background of your area of interest and find a problem or need. Following this, you can draft your background or Chapter 1.

Step 2: After you draft the background, you will complete a literature review.

Step 3: As you complete the literature review section, you will edit Chapter 1 which makes your case stronger.

The processes of reading literature and creating an OTD (occupational therapy doctorate) capstone project are intertwined, cyclical, and mutually beneficial. Students are able to identify a problem or need by gaining a thorough understanding of their area of interest, and the current state of practice through an examination of the literature. The identified problem or need then serves as the basis for the project type. Authors who have written on the topic and published in peer-reviewed journals act as virtual, informal mentors, steering the capstone project towards established problems. A successful capstone project not only draws from the existing body of knowledge, but also contributes to it.

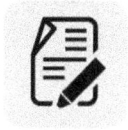

Worksheet 9.1: Getting Started

Modified from: Duncan, E. (2023). *Skills for Practice in Occupational Therapy.* Elsevier.

1. What do I currently know about the evidence for my area of interest?
2. On a scale from 1 to 5 how familiar am I with my area of interest?

Not familiar				Very familiar

3. How current is the literature I am reading?
4. After reviewing five articles related to my area of interest, what are three future implications or identified problems?

   1
   2
   3

5. On a scale from 1 to 5, how well do I understand the terms and concepts presented in these articles?

I don't under-stand many terms or concepts				I fully under-stand the terms and concepts

In the Beginning . . . Find a Way to Track Your Literature

For this section, please refer to the Literature Review Grid in Chapter 4.

As you start exploring literature relevant to your area of interest, find a way to keep track of your favorite articles. These favorite articles are ones you will reference throughout the background and literature review. To assist you in tracking literature in a meaningful way, this workbook provides a Literature Review Grid (see Chapter 4). This grid has categories to reduce the number of times you will need to re-read the original articles. By categorizing information the first time you read an articles, we hope for you to decrease the time needed to write different sections. However, the key is to review the categories of information to track and find a system that works for you.

MENU ITEM: BACKGROUND

If you are planning to write a background section to build your case, use the Learning Activities below.

Introduction

This section may include a guide to draft sections of a background that would create a compelling case to support a capstone project. While student projects will vary, we make suggestions for common themes to focus the writing at the paragraph level. If you would like to add more to the background section, there is flexibility in the paragraphs.

Now we'll talk about how to structure the information presented. The purpose of these guidelines is to help students write in a way that is structured for the reader. Use the advice of your doctoral coordinators and writing labs to help you effectively convey your thoughts and ideas as the writing process progresses. By breaking down each section into manageable chunks, this template can facilitate the writing process.

Suggested Order: Add or Modify Main Idea for Each Paragraph as It Fits with Your Area Of Interest

Paragraph 1: The introduction

Paragraph 2: The population

Paragraph 3: The larger problem – this is the larger problem influencing a population. At this level, the problem can be addressed by many stakeholders and practitioners.

Paragraph 4: The other professionals/interprofessional team that may be working towards improving the problem. What are the current services being offered to improve this challenge?

Paragraph 5: The role of occupational therapy. How can OT fill the gap between what is currently being done and the identified problem?

Paragraph 6: Theory, model, or frame of reference. What theory, model, or frame of refence will be used to support your project?

Paragraph 7: Conclusion (optional)

Writing the Background: Examples of Writing the Introduction to Chapter 1

Template for Introduction/Paragraph 1:

The purpose of this chapter is to convey the background evidence about the problem of _____. This chapter provides a background, problem, purpose, theory or model, significance, and rationale for the capstone project.

Example: Introduction A

First Draft of Introduction A:

The purpose of this chapter is to convey background evidence about the problem of occupational role dysfunction and decreased health outcomes for individuals in the ICU due to delirium. Occupational therapists can evaluate and treat to serve this population to improve role function and long-term outcomes for individuals in the ICU with delirium. This chapter provides a background, problem, purpose, significance, and rationale for the capstone project.

(Samantha M. – student sample)

Learning Activity 9.1: Improving the Sample

   1. How could the introduction be developed further?

   _____

   _____

   _____

   _____

---

2. How can you make this example better?

_____

_____

_____

_____

3. What strategies will you use when writing your introduction paragraph?

_____

_____

_____

_____

Example: Introduction B

Edited for the Final Submission:

The purpose of this chapter is to provide the reader with background knowledge on the diagnosis of congenital muscular torticollis – including statistics and definitions relevant to congenital muscular torticollis, client factors effected by this diagnosis, current treatment interventions – and describe what co-occupations are and how they are performed by caregivers and infants. This background section will describe the major issue that little is known about caregiver knowledge and adherence with the positioning of their infant diagnosed with CMT to optimize participation during co-occupations. A diagnosis of CMT in infancy puts increased demands and stress on caregivers, and limited caregiver knowledge and adherence with positioning infants with varying types and severities of CMT could lead to inadequate participation of the infants in co-occupations with the caregiver. The role of occupational therapy in the treatment of infants with congenital muscular torticollis and providing education to their caregivers will also be discussed. The Biomechanical Frame of Reference and Model of Co-Occupation will be used to justify how it guides this quantitative research type capstone project. (Dalton – student sample)

Learning Activity 9.2: Improving the Sample

1. How could the introduction be developed?

_____

_____

_____

2. How can you make this example better? Could it be synthesized?

_____

_____

3. What strategies will you use when writing your introduction paragraph?

_____

_____

_____

_____

Worksheet 9.2: Draft Your Introduction

Practice: Writing an introduction paragraph to your background section
Here is the template:
The purpose of this chapter is to convey the background evidence about the problem of _____ . This chapter provides a background, problem, purpose, theoretical model, significance, and rationale for the capstone project.

Main Idea Sentence

The purpose of this chapter is to convey the background evidence about the problem of

_____

_____

_____

_____

[What is your problem? _____].
Write 3–4 sentences that convey your message that includes the problem, purpose, significance, and rationale for the capstone project.

Paragraph 2: The Population

This refers to the population that is relevant to the capstone project. The goal is to provide statistics and definitions that will help a reader to better understand the characteristics of the chosen population. Letting your reader clearly understand the population is a way to introduce your area of interest.

Example: Paragraph 2

Sample: Children with ASD

Autism Spectrum Disorder (ASD) is a common developmental disorder that has been diagnosed with increasing frequency due to rising awareness of ASD symptomology. According to the Centers for Disease Control and Prevention (CDC), in 2014, the prevalence of children diagnosed with ASD is about 1 in 59 children, and males are about four times more likely to be diagnosed than girls (2019). ASD has been an area of interest to researchers and with more research being conducted, individuals are being diagnosed at a younger age than in the past. With the increase in diagnoses, research has led to the estimation of nearly half a million youth that will become adults in the next decade (Oswald et al., 2018). This is a large population of individuals in the community who will need to be able to be as independent as possible. (Courtney – student sample)

Learning Activity 9.3: Improving the Sample

1. How could paragraph 2 be developed?

_____

_____

_____

_____

2. How can you make this example better? Could it be synthesized?

_____

_____

_____

_____

3. What strategies will you use when writing your paragraph 2?

_____

_____

_____

_____

Worksheet 9.3: Draft Your First Paragraph

The main idea of this paragraph is to let readers know your population.

Sentence 1: Main idea sentence:

_____

_____

_____

Sentence 2: Evidence or supporting sentence:

_____

_____

_____

Sentence 3/4: Evidence or supporting sentence:

_____

_____

_____

Sentence 4/5: Concluding sentence:

_____

_____

_____

Paragraph 3: The Problem Affecting the Population

The main point of the paragraph is to communicate the problem or need influencing your population. To support this, several facts and statistics are provided to increase the reader's understanding of the problem at hand. The purpose of this paragraph is to raise awareness and understanding of the problem. By describing the problem concisely, readers will be able to see the relevance of your program and the role of OT in addressing the problem.

Example Paragraph 3:

Children in foster care are at a greater risk for mental health disorders such as ADHD, depression, anxiety, and other behavioral disorders (Engler et al., 2022). Instability and trauma are significant contributors to these disorders, as children in foster care frequently experience trauma prior to entering the system, and moving from home to home has been associated with higher rates of mental illness (Engler et al., 2022; Hindt and Leon, 2022). This instability and trauma also impair the child's ability to regulate their behavior and emotions, thereby limiting their participation in family, friendships, and school. Due to a lack of training in this area, foster parents have reported feeling ill-equipped to manage these complex behaviors (Hebert & Kulkin, 2018; Leffler & Ahn, 2022; Lotty et al., 2020; Kaasbll et al., 2019). This emphasizes the need for increased support and resources for foster children and foster parents. (Mackinzie)

Learning Activity 9.4: Improving the Sample

1. How could paragraph 3 be developed?

_____

_____

_____

_____

2. How can you make this example better? Could it be synthesized?

_____

_____

_____

3. What strategies will you use when writing your paragraph 3?

_____

_____

_____

_____

Practice Writing Paragraph 3 of the Background Section

The goal of this paragraph is to inform the readers about the larger challenge facing your population as a whole.

Sentence 1: Main idea sentence:

_____

_____

_____

_____

Sentence 2: Evidence or supporting sentence:

_____

_____

_____

Sentence 3/4: Evidence or supporting sentence:

_____

_____

_____

_____

Sentence 4/5: Concluding sentence:

_____

_____

_____

_____

Paragraph 4: What Is Currently Being Done?

The next one or two paragraphs have some variability. These paragraphs should help the reader to better understand the current state of the services attempting to address the issue impacting the population. In the following two paragraphs, we'll try to give you an in-depth look at the current state of services that are trying to fix a certain population's problem. OTs are not stand-alone professionals but rather part of a larger healthcare team. That's why we work hand-in-hand with other experts in the field to make the greatest possible difference for the people we help.

An OTD student should be able to describe the current context surrounding services for the population being served.

Example Paragraph 4

Current services provided in elementary schools for adolescents with disabilities include both special education and inclusive education, with the goal of implementing specially designed instruction that meets the needs of eligible students in the least restrictive environment at no cost to their parents (Hornby, 2021). IDEA requires school districts to develop transition plans for students when they are 16 years old, or as early as 14 years old in certain states. These plans outline action steps for achieving post-secondary transition goals in education, employment, independent living, and community participation (Pierce et al., 2021). As students transition from high school to postsecondary education, they are introduced to a new array of disability services offered by postsecondary institutions (Dragoo & Cole, 2019). Disability offices are frequently located on campus and are responsible for ensuring compliance with the Americans with Disabilities Act (ADA) and Section 504 in providing access to students with disabilities (U.S. Department of Education, n.d.). Despite the current services offered by teachers and post-secondary institutions, the transition outcomes for students with disabilities remain subpar.

NOTE: Here is where a gap is identified. This gap should be able to be filled by an occupational therapist and will be the focus of the OTD capstone project.

Learning Activity 9.5: Improving the Sample

1. How could paragraph 4 be developed?

_____

_____

_____

_____

2. How can you make this example better? Could it be synthesized?

_____

_____

_____

_____

3. What strategies will you use when writing your paragraph 4?

_____

_____

_____

_____

Practice Writing Paragraph 4 of the Background Section

The goal of this paragraph is to inform the readers about what is currently being done to address the problem.

Sentence 1: Main idea sentence:

_____

_____

_____

_____

Sentence 2: Evidence or supporting sentence:

_____

_____

_____

_____

Sentence 3/4: Evidence or supporting sentence:

_____

_____

_____

_____

Sentence 4/5: Concluding sentence:

_____

_____

_____

_____

Paragraph 5: What Is the Role of Occupational Therapy?

The purpose of this paragraph is to describe what is known that supports the role of the occupational therapist working with the population to fill the gap in the services being provided to the population. This paragraph should summarize why OT is the *best* profession to fill this gap and how OT can fill the identified gap better than another profession.

Example Paragraph 5

Occupational therapy is a profession that evaluates and treats young adults with ASD to improve social skills, behavior modification, and coping mechanisms to increase ability to find and keep employment. Despite the problems individuals with ASD have in these areas, OT services are frequently an unfunded service for young adults with ASD (Turcotte et al., 2016; van Schalkwyk & Volkmar, 2017). Therapists focus on aligning individuals' interests with job seeking and performance, as well as fostering active community, peer, and family engagement within these domains. Occupational therapists can address the problem by providing young adults with the skills necessary for successful long-term employment by implementing interventions such as work readiness, skill development, self-regulation strategies, and social participation (Hayward, McVilly, & Stokes 2019; Hedley et al., 2018).

   NOTE: Here is where a gap is identified. This gap should be able to be filled by an occupational therapist and will be the focus of the OTD capstone project.

Learning Activity 9.6: Improving the Sample

   1. How could paragraph 5 be developed?

   _____

   _____

   _____

   _____

   2. How can you make this example better? Could it be synthesized?

   _____

   _____

   _____

   _____

   3. What strategies will you use when writing your paragraph 5?

   _____

   _____

   _____

   _____

Practice Writing Paragraph 5 of the Background Section

The goal of this paragraph is to inform the readers about what is currently being done to address the problem.

Sentence 1: Main idea sentence:

_____

_____

_____

_____

Sentence 2: Evidence or supporting sentence:

_____

_____

_____

_____

Sentence 3/4: Evidence or supporting sentence:

_____

_____

_____

_____

Sentence 4/5: Concluding sentence:

_____

_____

_____

_____

Paragraph 6: What Theory, Model, or Frame of Reference Will Support Your Project?

This paragraph's goal is to explain the theoretical framework that will inform and direct your capstone project. This paragraph's main idea sentence identifies how a theory or set of theories will be applied to and relates to the capstone project. The subsequent sentences will elaborate and contextualize the main idea sentence by providing additional information that clarifies and supports the theoretical framework introduced in the main idea sentence. In addition, these sentences will summarize how the theory has been applied in similar contexts previously or how it could be applied in the present context. This paragraph's ultimate objective is to provide the reader with a comprehensive understanding of how the theory or theories shape and inform the project. The final sentence of the paragraph will restate the purpose of the paragraph and transition smoothly into the subsequent section of the project.

   Note: A common challenge during the drafting of this paragraph is students using the paragraph to teach others about the theory. This is NOT the purpose of the paragraph. This section applies a theory, model, or frame of reference to an OTD capstone project. The focus is the application of the theory, not a description of the theory.

Example Paragraph 6

The MOHO is the framework that can be applied to a research project exploring occupational role changes for survivors of intimate partner violence (Helfrich & Aviles, 2001). This model views individuals through a holistic lens, considering their environment as well as their roles, volition, and habits. According to Kielhofner (2008), these subsystems motivate, organize, and make possible occupational performance. More specifically, the MOHO provides insight into a survivor's performance and the contextual factors affecting their performance. This is important as the client's perspective on their situation is a precursor for change. An individual's environment may be assessed for potential risk, safety, and support systems. Roles include those from the person's past, present, and future; habits are addressed by examining the structure of an individual's day; and volition involves beliefs, values, interest, and sense of control (Kielhofner, 2008). Under MOHO, it is the responsibility of the occupational therapist 'to support client engagement in occupations in order to shape the client's abilities, their routine ways of doing things, and their thoughts and feelings about themselves' (Kielhofner et al., 2009, p. 448). Additionally, MOHO includes the notion that change in performance is achieved through occupational engagement, which refers to an individual's thought process and feelings while experiencing various situations in their environment. (Ikefuna – student sample)

Learning Activity 9.7: Improving the Sample

1. How could paragraph 6 be developed?

_____

_____

_____

_____

2. How can you make this example better? Could it be synthesized?

_____

_____

_____

_____

3. What strategies will you use when writing your paragraph 6?

_____

_____

_____

_____

Practice Writing Paragraph 6 of the Background Section

The goal of this paragraph is to inform the readers about what is currently being done to address the problem.

Sentence 1: Main idea sentence:

_____

_____

_____

_____

Sentence 2: Evidence or supporting sentence:

_____

_____

_____

_____

Sentence 3/4: Evidence or supporting sentence:

_____

_____

_____

_____

Sentence 4/5: Concluding sentence:

_____

_____

_____

_____

Paragraph 7: Conclusion

The goal of the final paragraph is to summarize and tie together the most important points made throughout the rest of the background section. Details about the population's demographics, gaps in care, service delivery, as well outcomes, theoretical underpinnings, and the value of occupational therapy are synthesized. The final sentence can state the capstone project's goal is to develop and implement a plan to improve these outcomes for the target population.

Example Paragraph 7

Young adults with ASD are faced with a disadvantage when it comes to gaining employment due to factors such as lack of social skills, self-determination skills, and support in the workplace (Baldwin et al., 2014; Rosales & Whitlow, 2019; Zalewska, Migliore, & Butterworth, 2016). Furthermore, 'in 2015, only 2% of autism research funds were directed towards adult issues,' indicating a need for this population (Anderson & Butt, 2018). In addition, another area that plays a role in job acquisition is the individual's stress-coping mechanisms (Oswald et al.,

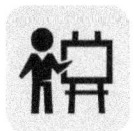

2018). An appropriate program for this population should be created to support employment and the transition from high school to adulthood (Chen et al., 2014). The significance of this capstone project is to develop an occupation-based program that will assist young adults with ASD with this transition period. (Courtney – student sample)

Learning Activity 9.8: Improving the Sample

1. How could the conclusion paragraph be developed?

_____

_____

_____

_____

2. How can you make this example better? Could it be synthesized?

_____

_____

_____

_____

3. What strategies will you use when writing your conclusion paragraph?

_____

_____

_____

_____

Practice Writing the Conclusion Sentence of the Background Section

The goal of this paragraph is to summarize key points from the entire background section.

Sentence 1: Main idea sentence:

_____

_____

_____

_____

Sentence 2: Describe what is being done:

_____

_____

Sentence 3/4: Describe how OT can improve on the problem:

_____

_____

_____

_____

Sentence 4/5: Identify the type of capstone project that will be developed to address the problem:

_____

_____

_____

_____

Writing the Problem Statement Section

In this section you will draft a paragraph to support your problem statement. This category of information is when you state your evidence-based problem or need. This section is the focus of the capstone project. This section provides a specific problem that is founded in current literature and is an existing problem.

Example Problem Statement Section

The problem is a lack of occupation-based programs addressing role competence for informal caregivers of individuals with SCI, resulting in caregiver burden and occupational imbalance (Jeyathevan et al., 2020; Zanini et al., 2020). There is a need to better integrate caregivers in the rehabilitation and discharge process to learn to take care of the health-related concerns and how to care for themselves in this new role. This is why the development of occupation-based programs are needed to educate individuals on their new role as an informal caregiver.

Studies have indicated that healthcare professionals, including occupational therapists, possess the necessary skills to design educational programs to counsel and prepare caregivers for their role, enabling them to provide optimal care and establish a healthy relationship with the patient after discharge. (Jeyathevan, et al., 2019). If caregivers can gain a sense of control and a full understanding of their role, they can decrease secondary complications associated with a spinal cord injury and cultivate a healthy relationship with their loved one, thereby limiting the overall burden and distress following the injury (Maitan et al., 2018). (Campisi – student sample)

Learning Activity 9.9: Improving the Sample

1. How could the problem statement section be developed?

_____

_____

_____

_____

2. How can you make this example better? Could it be synthesized?

_____

_____

_____

_____

3. What strategies will you use when writing your problem statement section?

_____

_____

_____

_____

Practice Writing the Problem Statement Section

The goal of this section is to summarize the key points about the problem in 1–2 paragraphs.

Sentence 1: The problem statement:

_____

_____

_____

_____

Sentence 2: Describe what is being done:

_____

_____

_____

_____

Sentence 3/4: Describe how OT can improve on the problem:

_____

Sentence 4/5: What is known about what could happen if the problem is resolved?

Writing the Purpose Statement Section

In this section you will draft a paragraph to support the purpose of the project to address the problem. In this section you will specify your project type, the goal of the project, and explain how the application of occupational therapy will address the problem. This section is the focus of the capstone project.

Example Purpose Statement Section

The purpose of this program development-type capstone project was to develop and facilitate an occupation-based program that focuses on health promotion, wellness, and prevention of obesity for children ages 9–12 to increase occupational engagement and health outcomes (Brockman et al., 2020; Schmalz et al., 2019). Occupational therapists are uniquely suited to address habit change by providing tools to promote occupational engagement in areas of health and wellness (Jessen-Winge et al., 2020). Multi-component interventions within community programming are recommended to influence and promote children's healthy habits and lifestyles (Weihrauch-Blüher & Wiegand, 2018). Occupational therapists can guide clients in developing healthy habits in their contexts to promote environmental change (Surrow et al., 2020).

There is a need for program development and piloted interventions to promote healthy habits such as healthy food options and meal preparation in after-school programs (Brockman et al., 2020). The 2021 AOTA statement indicates that OT practitioners are suited to deliver programs and services geared toward improving healthy behaviors by promoting healthy living practices, social participation, and occupational justice in healthy communities (Reitz et al., 2020). The proposed program development capstone project will implement an occupation-based program that will utilize OT practices and strengths in program creation to enhance and improve occupational engagement for children at risk for obesity. Therefore, the proposed capstone will evaluate the effectiveness of implementing an occupation-based program within a community setting for improved health outcomes. (Rodriguez – student sample)

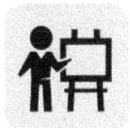

Learning Activity 9.10: Improving the Sample

1. How could the purpose statement section be better developed?

_____

_____

_____

_____

2. How can you make this example better? Could it be synthesized?

_____

_____

_____

_____

3. What strategies will you use when writing your purpose statement section?

_____

_____

_____

_____

Practice Writing the Purpose Statement Section

The goal of this section is to summarize key points about the purpose in 1–2 paragraphs.

Sentence 1: The purpose statement:

_____

_____

_____

Sentence 2: Describe how the purpose of your OT project improve on the problem:

_____

_____

_____

Sentence 3: What gap or need is filled by providing the OT project?

_____

_____

_____

Sentence 4: What is an overarching goal you want to achieve from your project?

_____

_____

_____

Learning Activity 9.11: Sample and Learning Activity

Understanding the goal of the background is to present information in a methodical way so the reader can understand your area of interest, the problem or need that exists, and what your project hopes to accomplish.

Practice analyzing a sample of the background section.

Chapter 1: Background

Sentence 1 – introduces population: In 2020, the Centers for Disease Control and Prevention (CDC) reported one in 54 children in America are diagnosed with autism spectrum disorder, affecting boys with a 4:1 ratio (Maenner et al., 2020).

Sentence 2–3 – Describes the focus of the problem for the population: Autism Spectrum Disorders (ASD) include an array of disorders characterized by early-onset impairments such as communicating difficulties in social situations and interacting with others and with restricted, repetitive interests and behaviors (Peretti et al., 2019).

Children with ASD experience difficulty with various tasks in their day-to-day lives such as generalization of tasks across different settings (de Marchena et al., 2015), social interactions with others (Peretti et al., 2019), speech and nonverbal communication (Franchini et al., 2018), and sensory processing (Kirby et al., 2017).

Last sentence – describes what will be coming in the rest of Chapter 1 background: Individuals with ASD can experience a number of co-occurring physical and mental health-related conditions such as seizures (Zhang et al., 2018), sleep disorders, attention-deficit/hyperactivity disorder (ADHD) (Romero et al., 2016), gastrointestinal disorders, feeding and/or eating challenges, obesity (Leader et al., 2020), obsessive compulsive disorder (OCD), anxiety (Romero et al., 2016), and depression (van Heijst et al., 2020).

Critique each sentence.

1. **Does the introductory sentence (sentence 1) of the paragraph introduce the population?**

   _____

   _____

   _____

   Could the sentence be written more concisely?

   _____

   _____

   _____

2. **Does sentence 2 focus the reader on a specific area of the population?**

_____

_____

_____

Could the sentence be written more concisely?

_____

_____

_____

3. **Does sentence 3 focus the reader on a specific area of the population?**

_____

_____

_____

Could the sentence be written more concisely?

_____

_____

_____

4. **Does the concluding sentence provide a conclusion to the paragraph and a potential link to the next paragraph?**

_____

_____

_____

Could the sentence be written more concisely?

_____

_____

_____

Learning Activity 9.12: Directions for Creating an Outline for an OTD Capstone Project

Background: Research and gather information about the population, gaps in outcomes and services and learn what the current evidence is about the challenges influencing your target population or problem. Create an outline for each potential paragraph to make the writing more efficient.

1. What is the population in one sentence?

_____

2. What are three references you will use to identify the population? Examples are prevalence, incidence, definitions. Governmental sources are good sources of statistics for this section. Expert tip: If you find descriptors on prevalence and incidence in the literature or from secondary sources, go to the referenced location. This way you will have the most current information available for your publication.

1

2

3

3. What is the problem? Chapter 5 provides details on the development of a problem statement. Prior to developing a final problem statement, you will have drafts of problems. Ultimately, the OTD capstone project focuses on a problem that can be addressed within a specific time frame.
The existence of the OTD capstone project is strong when the problem is supported by two current peer-reviewed references. Referencing and citing at least two current peer-reviewed references ensures that there are other experts in the field who would agree that the problem exists and that it is worth pursuing.
Problem: Clearly identify and describe the problem or issue that the project aims to address. Provide evidence to support the existence of the problem and its significance.
What are two potential problems you would like to address for your OTD capstone project?

1

2

4. What are the current services or solutions being used to address the problem?

1

2

3

5. What is the gap in the current services that results in the identified problem?

1

2

Worksheet 9.4: Peer/Self Feedback from Proposal/Background/AKA Chapter 1

Student submitting Chapter 1:_____

  Student providing peer guidance to Chapter 1: _____

Table 9.1 Peer/Self Feedback from Proposal/Background

	CONTENTS: Introduction, Background, Problem, Theory, Purpose, Rationale, Significance, and Definition of Terms	Peer Comments	Met/ Not Met Circle
	Editing Section 1		
The templates	Is the writing in the templates for your academic institution?		**Met/ Not Met**
The references	Are the references in APA – alphabetized, all have DOI, names of journals in italics?		**Met/ Not Met**
The references	Start with the references: Count how many current, peer-reviewed research articles there are to support the project. OPTIONAL: A *minimum* standard will be 30 articles supporting the project – 25 peer-reviewed, current research articles and 5 supporting/foundational articles. Most projects will have 50 or more articles– with 42 peer-reviewed, current articles and 8 supporting/foundational articles.	What is the total number of references?	**Met/ Not Met**
The references	OPTIONAL: To be current and peer-reviewed – look at the title of the article in relation to the population and problem, then look for the year of publication (must be less than 5 years from the graduation year), and then check the DOI.	Number of qualifying peer review articles:	**Met/ Not Met**
The references	OPTIONAL: There will be foundational literature, and some sources that are not research article for population statistics, but 85% (count how many you have) of the articles must be current (published less than 5 years from your date of graduation), Level 1 research articles.	Number of informational and educational references:	**Met/ Not Met**
The references	OPTIONAL: Are 85% of the references peer-reviewed?		**Met/ Not Met**
The references	Look at the titles of the articles – do the titles align with the focus of the project? Try to use current governmental statistics for population data versus textbooks or articles. References follow APA. Alphabetized, with DOI (use https://search.crossref.org/ to find DOIs).		**Met/ Not Met**
The references	As you read Chapter 1 – check off at each citation. Check – All citations are referenced.	Are all citations referenced? Be sure to let your peer know which ones are missing.	**Met/ Not Met**

Section 1 Met:
_____ /8

Editing Section 2

			Met/ Not Met
Background section Introduction	**Introduction:** 'The purpose of this chapter is to convey the background evidence about the problem of _____,_____. This chapter provides a background, problem, purpose, significance, and rationale for the capstone project. The chapter also includes planned objectives and deliverables for the experiential hour requirement of the capstone.	Is the header correctly formatted? Yes/No Does the introduction paragraph follow the writing guidance? Yes/No Does the introduction paragraph provide the reader with an understanding of the project? Yes/No	
Background section Paragraph 1	**Background:** Paragraph 1 (1 paragraph)– **describes the population.** Provide statistics and definitions relevant to the population. The Introduction paragraph: Sentence 1 (S1) (P1) – describe the main idea of the section. S2–4 – What are you going to be saying about the main idea? Last sentence – let the reader know what will be coming in the rest of this section (big problem, little problem, link to OT, and theory).	Does the first paragraph describe the population? Yes/No Is there a main idea sentence? Yes/No Are there supporting sentences that align with the main idea sentence? Yes /No	Met/ Not Met
Background section Paragraphs 2–3	**Paragraph 2–3 (1–2 paragraphs):** **Supporting details communicating a large/population level problem linked to the population.** Provide details, facts, examples, statistics, etc. that support the main idea Sentence 1: Main idea sentence/topic sentence – summarize the main point of the paragraph. Sentences 2–4: Supporting sentences – synthesize and support with citations information to increase the reader's depth of understanding with details about Sentence 1 Last sentence: Summarize the purpose of the paragraph and *transition to the next paragraph.*	Do the next two paragraphs communicate a problem relevant to the population described in paragraph 1? Yes/No Are there supporting sentences that align with the main idea sentence? Yes/No	Met/ Not Met

(Continued)

Table 9.1 (Continued)

CONTENTS: Introduction, Background, Problem, Theory, Purpose, Rationale, Significance, and Definition of Terms		Peer Comments	Met/ Not Met Circle
Background Final 3 paragraphs	**Paragraph 5–6 (1–2 paragraphs)Supporting details communicating how the problem is relevant to the profession of occupational therapy/the role of OT.** Provide details, facts, examples, statistics, etc. that support the main idea Sentence 1: Main idea sentence/topic sentence – summarize the main point of the paragraph. Sentences 2–4: Supporting sentences – synthesize and support with citations, information to increase the reader's depth of understanding with details about Sentence 1. Last sentence: Summarize the purpose of the paragraph and *transition to the next paragraph.* **Paragraph 7/ Last paragraph:** **Conclusion Paragraph:** Sentence 1: Main idea sentence/topic sentence – summarize the main point of the paragraph. Usually this restates the main idea of the section. Sentences 2–4: Supporting sentences – synthesizes and supports information from the section to support the claims made. Last sentence: Summarize the purpose of the paragraph and *transition to the next header.*	Is there a paragraph that has a main idea sentence, followed by supporting sentences that support how the problem is relevant to the profession of OT? Yes/No Is there a paragraph with a main idea sentence, followed by supporting sentences that clearly link a theory to the type of project and population? Yes/No Conclusion paragraph: Is there a conclusion paragraph that summarizes the previous paragraphs: population, relevant problem and issues, link to OT, and theory? Yes/No Are there adequate paragraphs to allow the reader to understand the background of the problem? Yes/No (If no – what area could be included?) Are there unnecessary/ repetitive paragraphs to allow the reader to understand the background of the problem? Yes/No (If yes – which paragraphs should be synthesized?)	Met/ Not Met

		Met/ Not Met
Editing for background section	Was this section easy to read? Yes/No Did each paragraph have a minimum of 5 sentences? Yes/No Did the sentences have no more than 15 words? Yes/No Did the sentences follow a noun, verb, adjective, prepositional phase formatting? Yes/No Were pronouns avoided? Yes/No	
		Section 1 Met: ___/5

Editing Section 3

		Met/ Not Met
Statement of the problem: A concise description of an issue to be addressed. (The problem has a larger problem. The problem statement demonstrates evidence of a clear problem that links to the profession, problem, and project.)	**Level 2 header:** **Problem statement:** S1: 'The problem is _____ _____ which results in (OR which is a problem because) _____' (Main idea sentence/topic sentence – Summarize the main point of the paragraph). Sentences 2–4: Supporting sentences – Synthesize and support with citations information to increase the reader's depth of understanding with details about Sentence 1. (*Ensure the problem is clearly stated and links to the purpose, project, and profession. There must be a minimum of 2 current peer-reviewed articles supporting that this is a problem.*)	Does the problem follow the template, clearly stating the problem? (Circle yes/no) 1. Does the first, main idea sentence state the problem? Yes/No 2. Is the first main idea sentence cited by at minimum of 2 references? Yes/No 3. As you scan the references, do you agree that the referenced authors would agree that the main idea sentence is a problem? Yes/No 4. Does the problem clearly link to the profession of OT? Yes/No
Purpose statement: clearly states what will be done to address the identified problem. (Project type is clearly stated; the purpose relates directly to problem, profession, and project; the outcome	**Level 2 header:** **Purpose statement** S1: 'The purpose of this (pick one: Program development/research/advocacy)-type capstone project is to (pick the one that aligns: Develop a program; qual. research= explore, quant. = analyze; advocate to) _____' (Main idea sentence/topic sentence – summarize the main point of the paragraph. Sentences 2–4: Supporting sentences – Synthesize and support with citations information to increase the reader's depth of understanding with	Does the purpose follow the template, clearly stating the purpose? (Circle yes/no) 5. Does the first main idea sentence state the purpose. Yes/No 6. Is the first main idea sentence clearly aligned with the problem statement? Yes/No

(Continued)

133

Table 9.1 (Continued)

CONTENTS: Introduction, Background, Problem, Theory, Purpose, Rationale, Significance, and Definition of Terms		Peer Comments	Met/ Not Met Circle
seems reasonable for the 14-week experience/hour requirement as is not too short or long).	details about Sentence 1. (*Ensure the purpose of the project is clearly stated, links to the problem, project, and profession.*) Last sentence: Summarize the purpose of the paragraph and *transition to the next paragraph or the next header.*	7. Does it seem reasonable to meet this purpose in 560 hours and 14 weeks? Yes/No 8. Does the purpose clearly link to the profession of OT? Yes/No 9. Does the purpose align with the recommendations of the literature? Yes/No	
Rationale: Clearly states why the project needs to be done. 1. What do you hope to contribute to the population of phenomena? 2. Why is this pursuit important? Answer the 'Who Cares about this project?' questions	**Level 2 header:** **Rationale** **P1:** S1: 'The rationale for this _____-type capstone project is to contribute to _____.' Sentences 2–3: Describe how the project will contribute to the population, profession, society, and other stakeholders. Last sentence: Summarize the purpose of the paragraph and *transition to the next header or paragraph.* **P2:** S1: 'This project is important because it will_____ _____.' OR 'The population will find this pursuit important because_____.' Sentences 2–3: Describe how the project is important to the population, profession, society, and other stakeholders. EDITING NOTE: This section has some variability as the main idea can be how the project contributes and is important to the population (P1), profession (P2), and society (P3.). Examples of 'other stakeholders' include – parents or teachers for a project that works with children; hospitals and other team members for a project that is focused on a system.	Does the rationale statement align with the formatting? Yes/No	**Met/ Not Met**

		Met/ Not Met
Significance: Clearly states what impact the project will have. A significance statement is a statement where the writer describes how the project will fill the gap identified by the problem statement. How does the project align with the problem? How will the project lead to positive change for the population or phenomena?	**Level 2 header: Significance** S1: 'The significance of the _____ _____-type project is it will fill the gap between _____ and _____.' Sentences 2–4: Supporting sentences describe how filling the gap aligns with the problem, purpose, and project. Last sentence: Conclusion.	Does the significance statement align with the formatting? Yes/No
Definition of terms	Are there terms that were not understood in the background? Yes/No (If no, there is no need for any definitions). Are there terms that were vague or needed further clarification? Yes/No (If yes – what terms? And they must be in the definition of terms). Are all terms cited? Yes/No	Met/ Not Met

REFERENCES

American Occupational Therapy Association (AOTA) (2014). Occupational Therapy Practice Framework: Domain and Process. *American Journal of Occupational Therapy, 68*(sup_1), S1–S48.

Dusick, D. (2014). Limitations and Delimitations of the Study. BOLD Educational Software. Retrieved from: http://bold-ed.com/barrc/assumptions.htm.

Hitzig, S. L., Jeyathevan, G., Farahani, F., Noonan, V. K., Linassi, G., Routhier, F., . . . & Craven, B. C. (2021). Development of Community Participation Indicators to Advance the Quality of Spinal Cord Injury Rehabilitation: SCI-High Project. *The Journal of Spinal Cord Medicine, 44*(sup_1), S79–S93.

Lai, H. Y., Tsai, L. L., & Lin, K. C. (2019). The Effectiveness of Telehealth in Occupational Therapy: A Systematic Review. *Journal of Telemedicine and Telecare, 25*(1), 3–9.

Literature Review

PIECING TOGETHER THE PROJECT PUZZLE: THE PROOF IS IN THE LITERATURE

A professional capstone paper is required in every program, whether it is an entry-level OTD or post-professional OTD. The main objective of the paper is to illuminate for the reader and clarify for the student the background of their capstone project (through a solid literature review), but also the gap discovered in the literature, with the ultimate chapters written telling the reader what happened and why during the capstone (methodology, implementation, discussion, conclusion).

In the development of the capstone paper, the literature review holds a unique position. This section is characterized by a love-hate relationship: Regardless of how frequently you find yourself summarizing and synthesizing literature, you will cherish the opportunity to share your synthesized insights and the knowledge supporting your project. Yet, the writing and editing process will always be a labor-intensive process that you may not enjoy.

The goal of the literature review is to examine current literature on a particular topic, and summarize and synthesize what is known about the concept. A literature review is more than just a summary or grouping of annotations; a literature review organizes and synthesizes these sources to offer a broader perspective. Remember:

- A summary condenses key points made from each source.
- A synthesis rearranges and/or reinterprets this information, potentially presenting a new perspective on old data, combining new and old interpretations, and comparing what is said between sources. A synthesis may also evaluate the quality and relevance of the sources and directs the reader to the most significant or relevant information.

THIS CHAPTER WILL GUIDE YOU THROUGH THE PROCESS OF WRITING A COMPREHENSIVE AND INSIGHTFUL LITERATURE REVIEW

Let's start with collecting and organizing the guest list. Who will be invited? Your invited guests are the articles you invite to your literature review party! But where should you start? Let's start with the problem that is your area of interest.

The problem is a lack of <u>occupation-based programs</u> **addressing role competence for informal caregivers** of *individuals with spinal cord injury, resulting in caregiver burden* and OCCUPATIONAL IMBALANCE (Guest 1: Jeyathevan et al., 2020; Guest 2: Zanini et al., 2020).

The two authors that would agree that this is a problem might be referenced many times throughout the literature review. They will be invited to many sections. What you will do next is find authors who analyze or explore each concept of the problem. How many articles you find can vary, but you want to read enough to develop an in-depth understanding of the concept.

Table 10.1 The Dinner Party

You have been invited to the dinner party hosted by *Summary or Annotation*

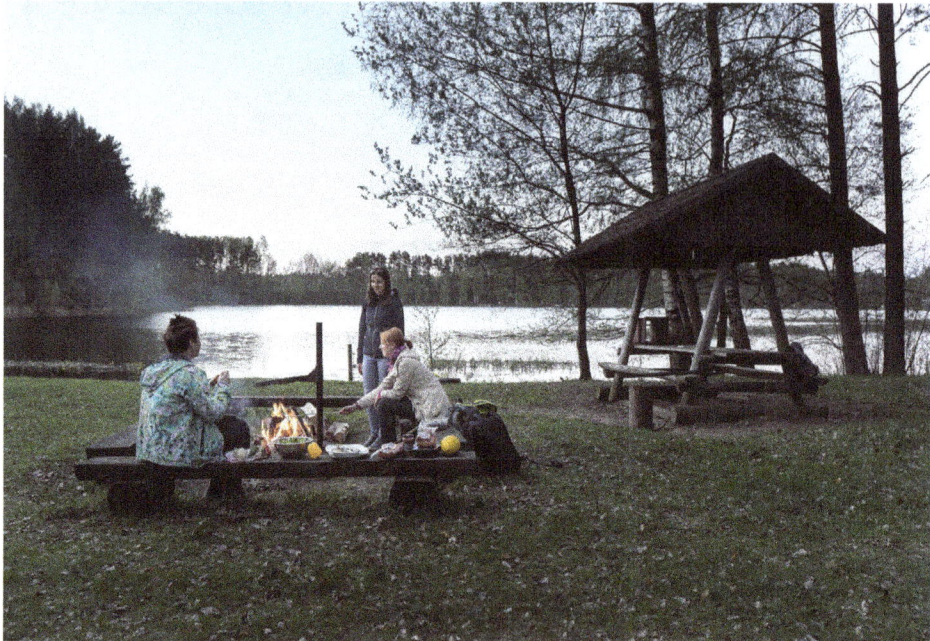

Figure 10.1 Dinner Party One Seating Arrangement Not Relevant

You have been invited to the Dinner Party Hosted by *Summary or Annotation*
All the guests have arrived. Appetizers have been served.

The host 'Summary' introduces each guest and then describes the contributions of each guest one at a time. Although their interests might overlap, there is no comparison. Only one guest's opinion is shared at a time.

You have been invited to the dinner party hosted by *Synthesis*

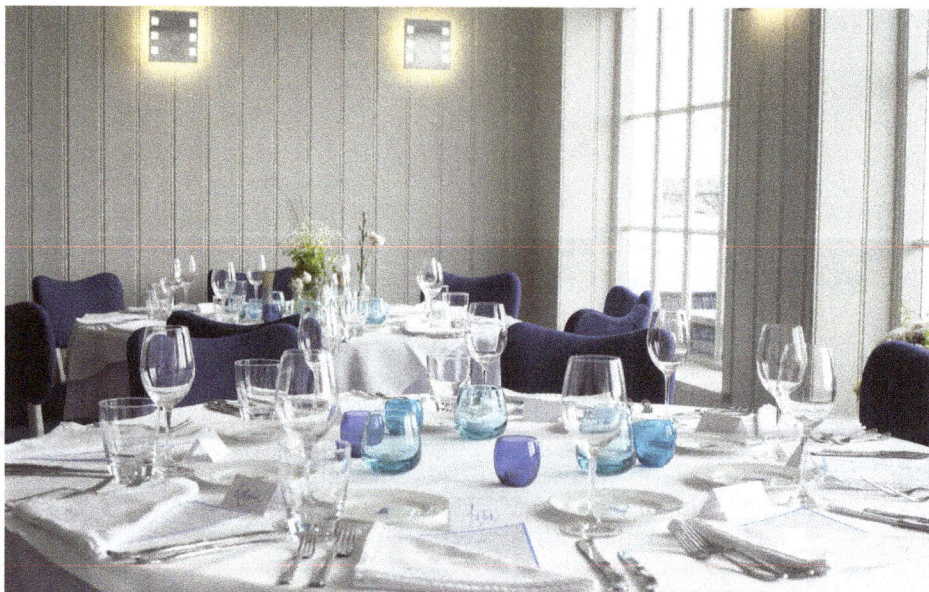

Figure 10.2 Dinner Party Two Seating Arrangement = Header/Theme/Concept

All the guests have arrived. Appetizers have been served.

The host 'Synthesis' has a seating arrangement where guests with similar interests are sitting together. The host introduces the guest as a group based on similarities and differences.

For example, Melissa and David both agree that individuals with post-concussion syndrome are under-diagnosed and are being diagnosed too late with post-concussion syndrome. David thinks this problem is due to the policies and procedures in emergency departments that limit referrals to rehabilitation. Melissa thinks this problem is due to limited healthcare providers on the interprofessional team.

A lively debate happens with other guests as to the similarities and differences in these findings. Could both be true? Could one be more relevant?

Jody interjects that she has found that occupational therapists, who already work in brain injury, can evaluate and treat individuals with post-concussion syndrome. Could this be a solution worth pursuing?

Comments that can be heard at Synthesis's party include:

'both authors *agree* that [point of agreement]' (Melissa, 2021; David, 2020)

Melissa (2021) states [] which *contrasts* with David's (2020) statement.

If the debate gets heated, the students can write specific differences, such as which author has a stronger case. For example:

Melissa's (2021) statement is stronger since her study was on 75 individuals with post-concussion syndrome, while David's was a single focus group.

Think of writing your literature review as hosting a 'dinner party.' Each article represents an esteemed guest. Depending on the number of concepts identified by your topic, you might host multiple such soirées. Start by introducing the topic to your readers, and then relay the insights and perspectives of your article guests. As the gracious host, remember that your role is to present their viewpoints without interjecting your own opinions. Your goal is to convey what your guests – the articles – have to share.

IN THIS EXAMPLE: SEARCH THE LITERATURE USING KEY TERMS FOR THESE CONCEPTS

- **addressing role competence for informal caregivers**
- *individuals with spinal cord injury*
- ***resulting in caregiver burden***
- OCCUPATIONAL IMBALANCE
- <u>evidence-based, occupation-based programs for SCI, caregivers, role competence for informal caregivers, and/or caregiver burden.</u>

Pro tip: Keep the literature categorized by concept. Either print and file each article by concept, or keep track of the concept in column 7 of the Literature Review Grid (see Chapter 4).

HOW MANY ARTICLES DO I NEED TO FIND?

There is no magic number for the number of articles per concept. As a general rule of thumb we suggest 8–10 articles.

If you have more than ten, then limit it down to your favorite, or most relevant articles.

If you have only two or three articles, that's not enough for a synthesis of a concept. Either keep searching, or combine that concept under a larger concept.

Pro tip: Keep the literature categorized by concept. Either print and file each article by concept, or keep track of the concept in column 7 of the Literature Review Grid (see Chapter 4).

Menu

What do you want to categorize on the Literature Review Grid?

- Article citation in APA
- What questions did the author ask or research?
- What are the key findings/summary/results of the article?
- What are the implications for the future?
- Overall evaluation of the article in relation to your capstone
- What type of study or methodological design is this?
- How does the article support your problem or project?
- Identify the theoretical or conceptual framework, model or theory
- Type of source or level of evidence
- For qualitative-type research, track and organize independent and dependent variables.

CONSIDERATIONS FOR TRACKING SPECIFIC INFORMATION

The following categories are examples of what you might put in a Literature Review Grid. Your college or university may have different suggestions. Reasons why these specific categories might be included are explained below:

1. Article citation in APA (or the format required by your academic institution). Citing the article in APA saves time and makes sure the references are used and cited correctly. Use this column to identify the article and to cut and paste with correct formatting.
2. What questions did the author ask or research? What was the purpose of the author's pursuit? (Usually found in the abstract). Identify what problem the authors were focusing on. Briefly summarizing the purpose of each article will help you understand the current societal issues that are being emphasized. Understanding the current state of knowledge prevents you from focusing on aspects of a problem that are already understood or have solutions.
3. What are the key findings/summary/results of the article? (Usually found in the abstract). Organizing an article's key findings, summaries, or results into a Literature Review Grid facilitates the categorization of current knowledge and consensus in the area of interest. This category lets you know your opportunities to build on what other people have found or if you should look in other directions.
4. What are the implications for future research identified by authors (creating a need)? (Usually found under discussion, implications for the future, or conclusion). Tracking and organizing implications for the future identifies trends in author recommendations to improve the problem. Students can be guided towards a project type by organizing the implications for the future stated in the articles. For instance, if multiple authors state there is a need for additional services and programs, this supports a need for a capstone project focused on program development. However, if the authors found there are effective programs, but the programs are not being implemented, this suggests the need for a leadership-based

capstone project focused on leadership strategies to overcome challenges to implementation.

5. Overall, personal, evaluation of the article in relation to your capstone (usually found in the abstract or conclusion). Including a statement of your favorite aspects of the article as it relates to your capstone project will help you figure out how the study relates to your area of interest. This makes sure that the literature you choose is relevant to your research goals and gives you useful information for your capstone project. Using the phrase: 'I liked this article because: _____' will help you keep track of the content and determine how you might use that content in your work later.

6. The type of article and methodological design. Identifying the type of study is important because it ensures you are looking at a wide range of literature. This workbook challenges you to include different kinds of studies, for example: three quantitative studies, three qualitative studies, one systematic review or meta-analysis, one book, and one international study.

Other options that could be included:

7. Identifying how this article supports your capstone project. State if you think the article relates to specific aspects of your project. For example, if you read an article and the problem appears related to the problem you want to address, write the word 'problem' in this column on the grid. Another example is if the article describes an advocacy plan that you might like to replicate, write 'purpose' in this column on the grid. If this category is complete, when writing a specific requirement, you can look at this column and separate out the categories that align with what you are writing at that time.

Additional categories might include:

1. Identify the theoretical or conceptual framework, model, or theory used. Categorizing the theoretical or conceptual framework can be helpful since this information gives the context of the research being done. You can choose to use the same theory or framework to support your capstone project.

2. Type of source or level of evidence. Tracking the type of source or level of evidence in a literature review is a meaningful practice for understanding the breadth, quality, and reliability of the information you are gathering. This category includes identifying if your source is a qualitative- or quantitative-type study, a book, an international article, or an opinion published in a peer-review journal. In addition to tracking the type of source, this category ensures a student doesn't inadvertently focus on only one type of source. For example, a student may inadvertently deviate towards reading only qualitative-type research articles. This might limit the understanding of what can be done quantitatively. A diverse assortment of source types contributes to a deeper and more thorough understanding of the area of interest.

3. For qualitative-type research, track the independent and dependent variables. Tracking the independent and dependent variables will help you to keep track of the key variables that are being studied. When it is time to synthesize the literature, you will be able to find which authors analyzed similar variables. Once you can see the variables in one spot, you can find patterns and trends in how different variables relate to each other. This is also helpful since you may want to use similar independent and dependent variables in your project.

4. For qualitative-type research, track and organize the data collection methods, reflexivity, and biases. Tracking the data collection method (i.e., focus group, interview, observation,) will help you to keep track of how data was collected to explore a topic. When it is time to synthesize the literature, you will be able to find which authors used similar techniques. Once you can see how the data was collected, you can make comparisons to see the type of understanding that was gained by the data collection method. This is also helpful since you may want to use similar data collection methods in your project.

5. The key terms used by the authors. Tracking the key terms identified in the literature you read is helpful since it helps you to understand the wording being used in the field. Tracking these terms allows you to identify and organize the terminology used by authors, so you can justify and use correct terminology. This tracking promotes clarity, rigor, and knowledge synthesis for the capstone project.

For this section, please refer to the Literature Review Grid in Chapter 4.

ORGANIZING YOUR THOUGHTS

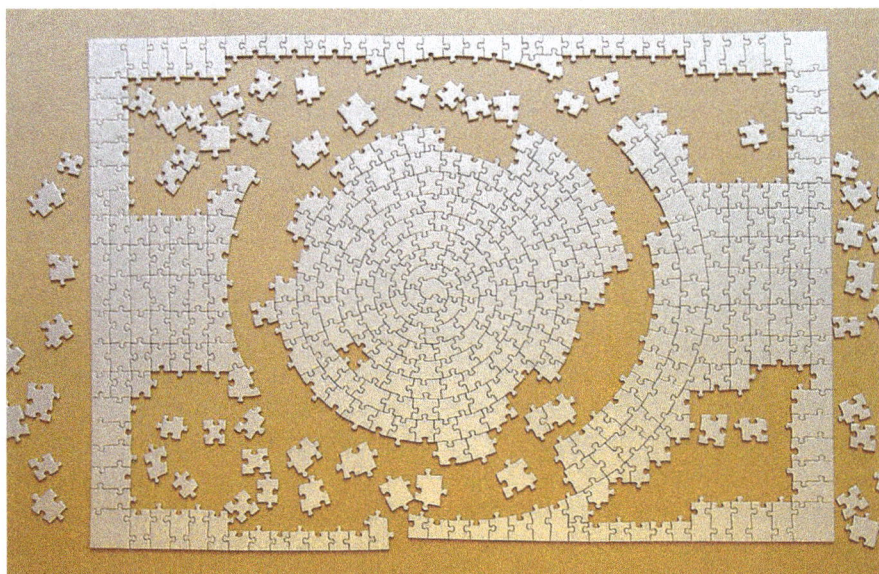

Figure 10.3 Jigsaw Puzzle

Use this as a mental image for planning to write a literature review.

The edges are the frame for your problem statement.

The piles of different colored pieces are the concepts learned while investigating the topic.

Each concept supporting the capstone topic resembles each pile of puzzle pieces, seemingly unrelated. The literature review synthesizes the concepts, much like putting together a puzzle, to provide a coherent picture of the topic at hand.

Once you have about 15 articles that align with your area of interest, across many of the concepts, you can start to draft a literature review.

Let's get started:

Example 1

Literature review or Chapter 2
Planning concepts to explore
Categorizing articles for each concept

1. **What is the problem or problem statement?**
   The problem is little is known about the perceptions of *individuals with upper limb amputations* **regarding the barriers to receiving prosthetic training and education** on prostheses advancements intended to decrease PROSTHESES ABANDONMENT and increase **occupational engagement** (Espinosa & Nathan-Roberts, 2019; Smail et al., 2021).

2. **What is the purpose or purpose statement?**
   The purpose of this qualitative research-type capstone project is to explore the perceptions of *individuals with upper limb amputations* **regarding the barriers they encounter to receiving prosthetic training and education** on prosthesis advancements intended to decrease PROSTHESIS ABANDONMENT and increase **occupational engagement** (Maza, 2023 – student sample).

3. **Identify key concepts/themes/headers from the problem and purpose statement.**
   Concept 1: *individuals with upper limb amputations*
   Concept 2: PROSTHESIS ABANDONMENT
   Concept 3: OPTIONAL but encouraged: Current services (to identify what is currently available)
   Concept 4: **barriers they encounter to receiving prosthetic training and education.** (Identifies a gap since current services still have these limitations)
   Concept 5: **occupational engagement**
   Concept 6: Role of OT to improve PROSTHESIS ABANDONMENT, **occupational engagement**
   Concept 7: Theory to support role of OT
   Conclusion

4. **Utilize columns 1 and 7 of the Literature Review Grid, OR categorize your literature to determine which articles provide insights into the key concepts, themes, or headers.**
   Theme/Header/Concept 1: *individuals with upper limb amputations*
   Theme/Header/Concept 2: PROSTHESIS ABANDONMENT
   Theme/Header/Concept 3: OPTIONAL but encouraged: Current services (to identify what is currently available)
   Theme/Header/Concept 4: **barriers they encounter to receiving prosthetic training and education** (identifies a gap since current services still have these limitations)
   Theme/Header/Concept 5: **occupational engagement**
   Theme/Header/Concept 6: Role of OT to improve PROSTHESIS ABANDONMENT, **occupational engagement**
   Theme/Header/Concept 7: Theory to support role of OT
   Conclusion

5. **Count how many articles you have relevant to the concept.**
   Concept 1: *individuals with upper limb amputations* – 10
   Concept 2: PROSTHESIS ABANDONMENT – 8
   Concept 3: OPTIONAL but encouraged: Current services (to identify what is currently available) – 6
   Concept 4: **barriers they encounter to receiving prosthetic training and education.** (Identifies a gap since current services still have these limitations) – 6

Table 10.2 Examples of Columns 1 and 7 of the Literature Review Grid

1	7
Article citation in APA	*What concepts were introduced or highlighted by this article? This section will help you pull relevant articles when writing each section of the literature review.*
Espinosa, M., & Nathan-Roberts, D. (2019). Understanding Prosthetic Abandonment. *Proceedings of the Human Factors and Ergonomics Society Annual Meeting, 63*(1), 1644–1648. https://doi.org/10.1177/1071181319631508.	*individuals with upper limb amputations* PROSTHESIS ABANDONMENT
Smail, L. C., Neal, C., Wilkins, C., & Packham, T. L. (2021). Comfort and Function Remain Key Factors in Upper Limb Prosthetic Abandonment: Findings of a Scoping Review. *Disability and Rehabilitation: Assistive Technology, 16*(8), 821–830.	*individuals with upper limb amputations* PROSTHESIS ABANDONMENT Current services **barriers they encounter to receiving prosthetic training and education**
Webster, J., Borgia, M., & Resnik, L. (2022). Prosthesis Nonuse and Discontinuation in United States Veterans with Major Limb Amputation: Results of a National Survey. *Prosthetics and Orthotics International*, 10–1097.	*individuals with upper limb amputations* PROSTHESIS ABANDONMENT Current services
Luza, L. P., Ferreira, E. G., Minsky, R. C., Pires, G. K., & da Silva, R. (2019). Psychosocial and Physical Adjustments and Prosthesis Satisfaction in Amputees: A Systematic Review of Observational Studies. *Disability and Rehabilitation: Assistive Technology, 15*(5), 582–589. https://doi.org/10.1080/17483107.2019.1602853.	PROSTHESIS ABANDONMENT Current services
Maxwell, J., Friedland, J., Kirsh, B., & Beaton, D. (2021). The Value Filter: A Novel Framework for Psychosocial Adjustment to Traumatic Upper Extremity Amputation. *Journal of Occupational Rehabilitation, 32*(1), 87–95. https://doi.org/10.1007/s10926-021-09976-5.	Theory to support role of OT Current services **barriers they encounter to receiving prosthetic training and education**
Law, M., Cooper, B., Strong, S., Stewart, D., Rigby, P., & Letts, L. (1996). The Person-Environment-Occupation Model: A Transactive Approach To Occupational Performance. *Canadian Journal of Occupational Therapy, 63*(1), 9–23. https://doi.org/10.1177/000841749606300103.	Theory to support role of OT
Romkema, S., Bongers, R. M., & van der Sluis, C. K. (2018). Influence of Mirror Therapy and Motor Imagery on Intermanual Transfer Effects in Upper-Limb Prosthesis Training of Healthy Participants: A Randomized Pre-Posttest Study. *PLOS ONE, 13*(10). https://doi.org/10.1371/journal.pone.0204839.	Current services
Resnik, L., Borgia, M., Ekerholm, S., Highsmith, M. J., Randolph, B. J., Webster, J., & Clark, M. A. (2021). Amputation Care Quality and Satisfaction with Prosthetic Limb Services: A Longitudinal Study of Veterans with Upper Limb Amputation. *Federal Practitioner, 38*(3), 110.	Current services **barriers they encounter to receiving prosthetic training and education**

Table 10.2 (Continued)

1	7
Grunert, B. K. (2020). Psychological Intervention with Upper Extremity Injured Patients in a Multidisciplinary Hand Center. *Journal of Health Service Psychology*, *46*, 81–87.	Current services **barriers they encounter to receiving prosthetic training and education**
Doroud, N., Fossey, E., & Fortune, T. (2015). Recovery as an Occupational Journey: A Scoping Review Exploring the Links Between Occupational Engagement and Recovery for People with Enduring Mental Health Issues. *Australian Occupational Therapy Journal*, *62*(6), 378–392.	*occupational engagement* – can be applied to amputee
Liu, Y., Zemke, R., Liang, L., & Gray, J. M. (2023). Occupational Harmony: Embracing the Complexity of Occupational Balance. *Journal of Occupational Science*, *30*(2), 145–159.	*occupational engagement* – can be applied to amputee
Nathan, E. P., & Winkler, S. L. (2019). Amputees' Attitudes toward Participation in Amputee Support Groups and the Role of Virtual Technology in Supporting Amputees: Survey Study. *JMIR Rehabilitation and Assistive Technologies*, *6*(2), 14887. https://doi.org/10.2196/14887.	Current services
Conceição de Maria, B., Galvão, C. R. C., & Carneiro, A. L. B. (2023). Interventions Used by Occupational Therapy in the Treatment of Amputees with Phantom Limb: An Integrative Review. *International Seven Journal of Health Research*, *2*(1), 26–58.	Role of occupational therapy
Crerar, E. (2023). Therapy and Rehabilitation in Maximizing Upper Extremity Amputation. *Operative Techniques in Orthopaedics*, 101062.	Role of occupational therapy Current services

Concept 5: *occupational engagement* – 2
Concept 6: Role of OT to improve PROSTHESIS ABANDONMENT, *occupational engagement* – 4
Concept 7: Theory to support role of OT – 2

6. **What concepts do you have enough literature to synthesize? (8–10 is a range)**

_____

_____

_____

_____

7. **What concepts do you need to gather more articles for to synthesize?**

_____

_____

_____

_____

Worksheet 10.1: Literature Review or Chapter 2

Planning Concepts to Explore: Categorizing Articles for Each Concept

1. What is the problem or problem statement?

_____

_____

2. What is the purpose or purpose statement?

_____

_____

3. Identify key concepts/themes/headers from the problem and purpose statement.

Concept 1:

Concept 2:

Concept 3:

Concept 4:

Concept 5:

4. Utilize columns 1 and 7 of the Literature Review Grid, OR categorize your literature to determine which articles provide insights into the key concepts, themes, or headers.

Table 10.3 Columns 1 and 7 of the Literature Review Grid

1	7
Article citation in APA	What concepts were introduced or highlighted by this article? This section will help you pull relevant articles when writing each section of the literature review.
_____	_____
_____	_____
_____	_____
_____	_____
_____	_____
_____	_____
_____	_____
_____	_____
_____	_____

_____

_____

_____

_____

_____

_____

5. Count how many articles you have which are relevant to the concept.

Concept 1: _____	Need more	Have Enough
Concept 2: _____	Need more	Have Enough
Concept 3: _____	Need more	Have Enough
Concept 4: _____	Need more	Have Enough
Concept 5: _____	Need more	Have Enough

Example 2

Synthesizing the literature per concept

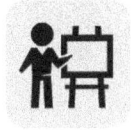

1. **Pick one of the concepts identified from Worksheet 10.1 (or the problem statement)**. Concept/Theme/Header: *individuals with upper limb amputations*
2. **List the articles (in APA) that provide an understanding of the concept**. If you have this identified in column 7 of the Literature Review Grid, then cut and paste that here.

Table 10.4 Example of Articles that Provide an Understanding of the Concept

Espinosa, M., & Nathan-Roberts, D. (2019). Understanding Prosthetic Abandonment. *Proceedings of the Human Factors and Ergonomics Society Annual Meeting*, *63*(1), 1644–1648. https://doi.org/10.1177/1071181319631508.	*individuals with upper limb amputations* PROSTHESIS ABANDONMENT
Smail, L. C., Neal, C., Wilkins, C., & Packham, T. L. (2021). Comfort and Function Remain Key Factors in Upper Limb Prosthetic Abandonment: Findings of a Scoping Review. *Disability and Rehabilitation: Assistive Technology*, *16*(8), 821–830.	*individuals with upper limb amputations* PROSTHESIS ABANDONMENT Current services **barriers they encounter to receiving prosthetic training and education**
Webster, J., Borgia, M., & Resnik, L. (2022). Prosthesis Nonuse and Discontinuation in United States Veterans with Major Limb Amputation: Results of a National Survey. *Prosthetics and Orthotics International*, 10 1097.	*individuals with upper limb amputations* PROSTHESIS ABANDONMENT Current services

3. **Gather the articles and identify the most important concepts you want to share with your reader.**

   a. Define upper limb amputation
   b. Provide incidence, etiology, and prevalence
   c. Describe physical and mental impairments post-amputation
   d. Describe upper extremity prosthetics and rehabilitation.

4. **Draft a main idea sentence for the first paragraph**.

A good idea is to start the main idea sentence with the concept in the sentence. In this case: *individuals with upper limb amputations.*

Main idea sentence: Upper limb amputation entails the surgical removal of any portion of the upper extremity, whether because of surgical needs, unique trauma, or disease.

Then draft a 3–5 paragraph synthesis of the selected articles:

An upper limb amputation is the surgical removal of any part of the upper extremity due to surgery, trauma, or pathology. Upper limb removal can consist of any part of the arm, forearm, hand, and digits. The leading cause of upper limb amputations is trauma which more commonly occurs in males aged 15–25 years old (Maduri & Akhondi, 2023). Approximately 300 to 500 new amputations occur daily (Lee et al., 2022). The most common mechanism is motor vehicle collisions.

The general principles of upper extremity amputation will be common to all types of amputations. The goal is to remove a distal segment of the extremity, meaning there is a need to divide and realign all the structures which include the arteries, veins, nerves, tendons, ligaments, and bones will have to be divided (Ovadia and Askari, 2015). Preservation of extremity length is often a goal for the individual but that depends on the severity of the limb amputation. It is more beneficial for the individual to have a longer limb rather than a shorter one.

There are different levels of upper-limb amputation, the first one being shoulder disarticulation, which is at the shoulder. The second one is transhumeral which is above the elbow. Elbow disarticulation is located at the elbow. Transradial is located below the elbow. Wrist disarticulation is at the wrist and partial hand which includes fingers and any part of the hand. Each level of amputation is different and has its own implications and limitations (Espinosa & Nathan-Roberts, 2019).

Physically, the body must adjust to the loss of a limb, deal with phantom limb pain, and train functional skills with the artificial limb to perform activities at work or other activities of daily living (Luza et al., 2019). Despite the large and increasing number of individuals living with limb loss, current rehabilitation strategies, including prosthetic training, are often inadequate and unstandardized due to a lack of evidence to guide clinical practice (Lee et al., 2022).

After amputation, the rehabilitation process, and the use of an artificial limb that allows individuals to maintain their mobility and independence tend to improve their physical and mental well-being (Luza et al., 2019). The rehabilitation process needs to begin right after amputation so that individuals adapt to the new condition they're living with and begin using an artificial limb to participate in their everyday tasks. The artificial limb offers amputees a fresh opportunity to perform the function that would have been performed by the missing body part (Brack & Amalu, 2021; Maza, 2023 – student sample).

Worksheet 10.2: Synthesizing the Literature per Concept

1. Pick one of the concepts identified from Worksheet 10.1 (or the problem statement).

Concept/Theme/Header

2. List the articles (In APA) that provide an understanding of the concept. (If you have this identified in column 7 of the Literature Review Grid, then cut and paste that here):

1

2

3

4

5

6

7

8

9

10

3. After reviewing the selected articles, identify the most important concepts to share with your reader.

1

2

3

4

4. Draft a main idea sentence for the first paragraph:

_____

_____

5. Draft a 3–5 paragraph synthesis of the selected articles.

_____

_____

_____

_____

_____

_____

_____

_____

_____

_____

_____

_____

_____

_____

_____

_____

_____

Conclusion

To write each section, header, or theme, use Worksheets 10.1 and 10.2 for each concept.

It goes beyond the scope of this workbook to teach writing skills at the sentence or paragraph level. If you have concerns about your writing, search for resources on writing a five-paragraph essay so you can find examples; or approach your academic institution, who will have writing center support. One method of paragraph writing that aligns well with the writing style used for a literature review is the MEAL plan style (see Duke University, n.d.). Begin each paragraph with a **M**ain idea sentence, then the **E**vidence, **A**nalysis and then **L**ink the paragraph to the rest of the section. Using this format makes it easier for the reader to follow the written concepts being conveyed.

As you write and edit, imagine the process of writing a literature review as filling in all the pieces of the puzzle. Each concept, representing various sources and insights, fits together seamlessly to reveal a complete picture of your capstone topic.

FREQUENTLY ASKED QUESTIONS

1. **What is the purpose of Chapter 2 or literature review in a capstone project?** The purpose of the literature review is to demonstrate the relevance and necessity of your project in the context of current research. The writing of a literature review establishes a foundation for your research, identifies gaps, and justifies the necessity of your study. Reading a literature review provides the reader with an understanding of the current context surrounding your area of interest.

2. **What is the best method to develop a literature review?** There is no best method for developing a literature review; it is an iterative process rather than a one-size-fits-all approach (Paré & Kitsiou, 2017). Writing a literature review involves progressively reading and integrating literature to build a solid foundation for your area of interest. The literature is organized into coherent categories, helping readers grasp the current state of knowledge around your topic. The way the literature is categorized presents a clear picture of the existing situation and demonstrates your ability to use evidence-based practices in guiding the development of your capstone project. (Paré & Kitsiou, 2017).

3. **How should I organize my review of the relevant literature?** There is no best method for organizing the themes or headers for a literature review (Paré & Kitsiou, 2017). To provide guidance, this workbook suggests grouping your literature into sections (aka themes or headers) that align with specific aspects of your area of interest. Common themes for many student projects include sections on:

   a. The target population
   b. The problem being addressed
   c. Current services available

d. The role of occupational therapy

e. The theoretical framework guiding the project.

Given the time constraints typical of a capstone project, organizing your literature review around these themes meets the purpose of a literature review. However, depending on the specifics of your project, other relevant themes might include:

a. Economic impact of the issue

b. Societal impact

c. Political influences

d. Comparative analysis of local, state, national, and international efforts to address the issue

Organizing your literature into groups of 8–10 pieces of current literature, and synthesizing these articles into a theme allows the student a strategy to develop a comprehensive literature review.

4. **What steps should I take to avoid plagiarism?** Avoiding all forms of plagiarism goes beyond the scope of this workbook. You must give credit to original authors by citing them in the appropriate format used by your academic institution. Make use of tools that check for plagiarism, and ensure you follow the citation guidelines established by your educational institution.

5. **How do I incorporate studies that contradict each other into my literature review?** You should point out studies that contradict one another because doing so demonstrates you have a comprehensive understanding of the subject matter. Clearly stating differences in what is known about an issue brings attention to the complexity and variety of perspectives that exist within the field. Reading articles and then pointing out areas of agreement and disagreement provides you with an in-depth understanding of you area of interest.

6. **How long should my literature review be?** This is the most common question we get! There is no set length for a literature review (Paré & Kitsiou, 2017). The length of a literature review is determined by the significance of the subject matter as well as the requirements of the academic program that you are enrolled in.

To provide guidance, this workbook suggests grouping your literature into sections (aka themes or headers) that align with specific aspects of your area of interest. Each theme would be supported by 8–10 pieces of current literature. These articles may overlap. Table 10.5 shows estimates of the length for a literature review.

Table 10.5 Estimated Length for a Literature Review

Sample Header or Theme	Number of Articles	Header Length	Pages
The target population	8–10	8–10 articles synthesized into approximately a 4–5 paragraph essay.	650–1100 words or 3–4 pages, double spaced
The problem being addressed	8–10	8–10 articles synthesized into approximately a 4–5 paragraph essay.	650–1100 words or 3–4 pages, double spaced
Current services available to address the problem (tends to end with the gap in current services/situation)	8–10	8–10 articles synthesized into approximately a 4–5 paragraph essay.	650–1100 words or 3–4 pages, double spaced

(Continued)

Table 10.5 (Continued)

The role of occupational therapy (tends to support how OT can fill the gap in current services)	8–10	8–10 articles synthesized into approximately a 4–5 paragraph essay.	650–1100 words or 3–4 pages, double spaced
The theoretical framework guiding the project	4–6	4–6 articles synthesized into approximately a 2–3 paragraph essay	350–650 words or 2–3 pages double spaced
Total	36–46 articles (some articles will be synthe-sized in more than one header)	5 headers or themes, 18–23 paragraphs	2,950–5,050 words, or 12–19 pages double spaced.

Source: Data modified from Academic Marker, 2022.

REFERENCES

Academic Marker (2022, April 25). What are the Six Different Essay Lengths? Retrieved from: https://academicmarker.com/academic-guidance/assignments/essays/what-are-the-six-different-essay-lengths/.

Brack, R., & Amalu, E. H. (2021). A Review of Technology, Materials and R&D Challenges of Upper Limb Prosthesis for Improved User Suitability. *Journal of Orthopaedics*, *23*, 88–96.

Conceição de Maria, B., Galvão, C. R. C., & Carneiro, A. L. B. (2023). Interventions Used by Occupational Therapy in the Treatment of Amputees with Phantom Limb: An Integrative Review. *International Seven Journal of Health Research*, *2*(1), 26–58.

Crerar, E. (2023). Therapy and Rehabilitation in Maximizing Upper Extremity Amputation. *Operative Techniques in Orthopaedics*, 101062.

Doroud, N., Fossey, E., & Fortune, T. (2015). Recovery as an Occupational Journey: A Scoping Review Exploring the Links Between Occupational Engagement and Recovery for People with Enduring Mental Health Issues. *Australian Occupational Therapy Journal*, *62*(6), 378–392.

Duke University (n.d.). Paragraphing: The MEAL Plan. Retrieved from: https://twp.duke.edu/sites/twp.duke.edu/files/file-attachments/meal-plan.original.pdf.

Espinosa, M., & Nathan-Roberts, D. (2019). Understanding Prosthetic Abandonment. *Proceedings of the Human Factors and Ergonomics Society Annual Meeting*, *63*(1), 1644–1648. https://doi.org/10.1177/1071181319631508.

Grunert, B. K. (2020). Psychological Intervention with Upper Extremity Injured Patients in a Multidisciplinary Hand Center. *Journal of Health Service Psychology*, *46*, 81–87.

Jeyathevan, G., Cameron, J. I., Catharine Craven, B., Munce, S. E. P., & Jaglal, S. B. (2019). Re-building Relationships After a Spinal Cord Injury: Experiences of Family Caregivers and Care Recipients. *BMC Neurology*, *19*(1), 1–13. https://doi.org/10.1186/s12883-019-1347-x.

Jeyathevan, G., Catherine Craven, B., Cameron, J. I., & Jaglal, S. B. (2020). Facilitators and Barriers To Supporting Individuals with Spinal Cord Injury in the Community: Experiences of Family Caregivers and Care Recipients. *Disability and Rehabilitation*, *42*(13), 1844–1854. doi:10.1080/09638288.2018.1541102.

Law, M., Cooper, B., Strong, S., Stewart, D., Rigby, P., & Letts, L. (1996). The Person-Environment-Occupation Model: A Transactive Approach To Occupational Performance.

Canadian Journal of Occupational Therapy, *63*(1), 9–23. https://doi.org/10.1177/000841 749606300103.

Lee, S. P., Bonczyk, A., Dimapilis, M. K., Partridge, S., Ruiz, S., Chien, L. C., & Sawers, A. (2022). Direction of Attentional Focus in Prosthetic Training: Current Practice and Potential for Improving Motor Learning in Individuals with Lower Limb Loss. *PLOS One*, *17*(7), e0262977.

Liu, Y., Zemke, R., Liang, L., & Gray, J. M. (2023). Occupational Harmony: Embracing the Complexity of Occupational Balance. *Journal of Occupational Science*, *30*(2), 145–159.

Luza, L. P., Ferreira, E. G., Minsky, R. C., Pires, G. K., & da Silva, R. (2019). Psychosocial and Physical Adjustments and Prosthesis Satisfaction in Amputees: A Systematic Review of Observational Studies. *Disability and Rehabilitation: Assistive Technology*, *15*(5), 582–589. https://doi.org/10.1080/17483107.2019.1602853.

Maduri, P., & Akhondi, H. (2023). Upper Limb Amputation. In: *StatPearls* [Online]. StatPearls Publishing. Retrieved from: https://www.ncbi.nlm.nih.gov/books/NBK540962/.

Maxwell, J., Friedland, J., Kirsh, B., & Beaton, D. (2021). The Value Filter: A Novel Framework for Psychosocial Adjustment to Traumatic Upper Extremity Amputation. *Journal of Occupational Rehabilitation*, *32*(1), 87–95. https://doi.org/10.1007/s10926-021-09976-5.

Nathan, E. P., & Winkler, S. L. (2019). Amputees' Attitudes toward Participation in Amputee Support Groups and the Role of Virtual Technology in Supporting Amputees: Survey Study. *JMIR Rehabilitation and Assistive Technologies*, *6*(2), 14887. https://doi.org/10.2196/14887.

Ovadia, S. A., & Askari, M. (2015, February). Upper Extremity Amputations and Prosthetics. *Seminars in Plastic Surgery*, *29*(1), 55–61.

Paré, G., & Kitsiou, S. (2017). Methods for Literature Reviews. In *Handbook of eHealth Evaluation: An Evidence-based Approach* [Online]. University of Victoria.

Resnik, L., Borgia, M., Ekerholm, S., Highsmith, M. J., Randolph, B. J., Webster, J., & Clark, M. A. (2021). Amputation Care Quality and Satisfaction with Prosthetic Limb Services: A Longitudinal Study of Veterans with Upper Limb Amputation. *Federal Practitioner*, *38*(3), 110.

Romkema, S., Bongers, R. M., & van der Sluis, C. K. (2018). Influence of Mirror Therapy and Motor Imagery on Intermanual Transfer Effects in Upper-Limb Prosthesis Training of Healthy Participants: A Randomized Pre-Posttest Study. *PLOS ONE*, *13*(10). https://doi.org/10.1371/journal.pone.0204839.

Smail, L. C., Neal, C., Wilkins, C., & Packham, T. L. (2021). Comfort and Function Remain Key Factors in Upper Limb Prosthetic Abandonment: Findings of a Scoping Review. *Disability and Rehabilitation: Assistive Technology*, *16*(8), 821–830.

Treisman, H., Ratzon, N. Z., Itzkovich, M., & Avrech Bar, M. (2020). Performance of Everyday Occupations and Perceived Health of Spouses of Men with Spinal Cord Injury at Discharge and 6 Months Later. *Spine*, *45*(22), 1580–1586. http://dx.doi.org/10.1097/BRS.000000 0000003630.

Webster, J., Borgia, M., & Resnik, L. (2022). Prosthesis Nonuse and Discontinuation in United States Veterans with Major Limb Amputation: Results of a National Survey. *Prosthetics and Orthotics International*, 10–1097.

Zanini, C., Fiordelli, M., Amann, J., Brach, M., Gemperli, A., & Rubinelli, S. (2020). Coping Strategies of Family Caregivers in Spinal Cord Injury: A Qualitative Study. *Disability and Rehabilitation*, *44*(2), 243–252. doi:10.1080/09638288.2020.1764638.

11

Blueprints to Brilliance: Crafting Your Capstone Plan
Writing Objectives for Your Capstone Project

THE PROJECT PLAN, METHODOLOGY, AND WRITING PROJECT OBJECTIVES SYNONYMOUS WITH CHAPTER 3

After reviewing the literature, conducting a needs assessment, defining the specific problem, and selecting the type of project, it's now time to draft your project plan. This section serves as a road map, outlining how you intend to bring your project from your concept to completion. Keep in mind that the purpose of this section is not simply to present a plan, but also to demonstrate to your doctoral coordinator and others that the project is viable. By the end of Chapter 3, your reader should be confident in your project's direction and your ability to execute it within the stipulated time frame.

To navigate this process successfully, you will:

1. **Articulate your capstone project vision:** Begin by giving an overview of your intended capstone project. This is the 'what' of your project – i.e., the project you hope to complete.
2. **Outline your approach:** Here, you will describe the procedures or methods you will employ. Consider this the 'how' – the techniques, tools, and strategies you intend to use to complete the project.
3. **Develop a project timeline:** Here is where you will draft a practical timeline that ensures your objectives are met within the allotted time frame. It is essential to be practical and to allow for flexibility.
4. **Create a measurement or deliverable:** Determine how you will evaluate the project objective outcomes and determine the project's success. Determine what method you will use to highlight the project's successes and areas for improvement.
5. **Ensure depth and specificity:** Each step should be described in sufficient detail to demonstrate both its viability and your preparedness. A well-considered plan demonstrates your dedication to the project and explains how you will show the project has been completed.

Table 11.1 Examples for Capstone Project Objectives (POs)

Clinical Practice Skills	1. Get approvals for the plan of specific clinical practice skill(s) to be implemented
	2. Recruit clients or relevant individuals
	3. Track provision of clinical practice skills in alignment with the plan
	4. Monitor the outcomes
	5. Complete quality assurance measures with clients and supervisors or mentors
	6. Publish or present a clinical pathway describing the guidelines for best practice implementation of the clinical practice skill(s).

(Continued)

Table 11.1 (Continued)

Research Type	1. Complete IRB (institutional review board; ideally, this should be completed before the start of the experience) 2. Recruit participants 3. Collect data 4. Evaluate data 5. Publish or present data.
Administration	There are common threads in project types between administration and leadership. For these examples, administration is at a group or departmental level. 1. Get approvals for the planned objective type. For example: Workflow metrics, staff training system development, resource allocation, burnout prevention 2. Implement the planned objective 3. Track progress 4. Complete a quality assurance plan 5. Publish or present on the project outcomes.
Leadership	There are common threads in project types between administration and leadership. For these examples, leadership is at an organizational level. 1. Disseminate the planned objective type. For example: Strategic growth planning; diversity, equity and inclusion initiatives; conflict resolution; analysis of legal, fiscal, or regulatory factors; organizational effectiveness initiatives 2. Implement the planned objective 3. Track progress 4. Complete a quality assurance plan 5. Publish or present on the project outcomes.
Program and Policy Development	1. Develop a program (ideally, this is started before the start of the experience) 2. Implement the program 3. Track progress 4. Complete a quality enhancement plan 5. Develop a policy for sustainability for the program 6. Publish or present on the program and policy outcomes.
Advocacy	1. Identify what you will be advocating and to whom. For example: Community or facility leadership, government officials, social media, civic groups, non-profit leadership, or stakeholders relevant to your area of interest 2. Conduct stakeholder analysis and engagement planning 3. Develop a clear message and communication strategy 4. Implement the outreach plan 5. Monitor progress 6. Develop a sustainability plan for the project. 7. Publish or present on the advocacy outcomes.
Education	1. Identify the gap in knowledge for a specific population/audience 2. Design the curriculum, objectives, and course outlines 3. Develop the educational modules, training sessions, or continuing education units (CEU) 4. Schedule the education session(s) 5. Track participant progress 6. Develop a sustainability plan for the educational module(s) 7. Publish or present on the educational outcomes.

Table 11.1 (Continued)

Theory Development	Note: Theory development can overlap with all other project types.
	1. Determine the stage of development or need for advancement for a particular framework, model, or theory. Or determine the need to apply a known framework, model, or theory to a new population.
	2. Identify and collaborate with authors, mentors, and scholars who have made notable contributions to the framework, model, or theory.
	3. Devise a strategy either to enhance the framework, model, or theory, or to implement it specifically for a target population.
	4. Develop a sustainability plan for continued development of the framework, theory, or model.
	5. Present or publish new hypotheses, redefining concepts, suggesting new relationships, or emphasizing potential applications to the target population and/or authors, mentors, and scholars.

Worksheet 11.1: Mission: Capstone – From Vision to Timeline: Developing the Project Timeline with Deliverables

Use this worksheet as a road map to organize your thoughts, approaches, and plans to develop a capstone project, and to think critically about feasibility.

1. In simple terms, what is your vision for the capstone project? If you haven't decided, pick one of the project types and state what you will do to address the problem using this project type.

a. Identify the main objective of your capstone project in one sentence.

b. List 1–3 key outcomes that you expect from your project upon its completion.

1

2

3

c. Using Figure 1: Template of project objectives, modify these sample objectives to align with your project.

Objective 1

Objective 2

Objective 3

Objective 4

Objective 5

2. Outline your strategy:

a. Identify and list the primary methods and/or techniques that will be utilized to meet the objective for the project.
b. Document the tools and resources required to complete the project.
c. Describe any potential obstacles you anticipate and how your chosen strategies will address them.

3. Draft a project schedule:

a. Divide your project into major milestones and assign each one a tentative due date and approximate amount of time in the grid below. Include buffer time in your timeline for unforeseen delays or obstacles.
b. Evaluate your schedule. Which steps would need support from your mentor? Are there any steps that may require additional time? Are there any overlapping or concurrent steps? Adjust as necessary.

Table 11.2 Project Schedule

Week/ insert date	*What project objective will be addressed?* *There are weeks where there will be no time dedicated to a project objective as you will be at your experience.*	*Comments: How long will this step take? Do you need support from others/mentors to achieve this step?*
Week 1		
Week 2		
Week 3		
Week 4		
Week 5		
Week 6		
Week 7		
Week 8		
Week 9		
Week 10		
Week 11		
Week 12		
Week 13		
Week 14		

Note: Total hours dedicated to project: 40–45 hours over 14 weeks.

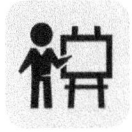

Worksheet 11.1 Example: Mission: Capstone – From Vision to Timeline

Use this worksheet as a road map to organize your thoughts, approaches, and plans to develop a capstone project, and to think critically about feasibility.

1. **In simple terms, what is your vision for the capstone project? If you haven't decided, pick one of the project types and state what you will do to address the problem using this project type.**

   a. Identify the main objective of your capstone project in one sentence.
   I want to research occupational therapist evaluation and intervention to help the obesity epidemic.

   b. List 1–3 key outcomes that you expect from your project upon its completion.
   I want to develop a research-type project where I learn about challenges that occupational therapists have working with children with obesity.
   I think I will learn about occupational performance deficits for children with obesity.

   c. Using Figure 1: Template of project objectives, modify these sample objectives to align with your project.
   Objective 1: Complete IRB (ideally, complete before the start of the experience). I plan to work with the DCC to complete IRB before starting the experience.
   Objective 2: Recruit participants: After IRB approval I will post my flyer at (location) to recruit participants to complete the Pizzi Healthy Weight Management Assessment.
   Objective 3: Collect data. As I get participants, I will complete the assessment and record the data.
   Objective 4: Evaluate data. After all the data is collected, I will analyze the data.
   Objective 5: Publish or present data. I will present the data at my university poster presentation.

2. **Outline your strategy:**

   a. Identify and list the primary methods and/or techniques that will be utilized to meet the objective for the project.
   I will use a qualitative methodology to collect data. I will use Google Forms to input the findings electronically.

   b. Document the tools and resources required to complete the project.
   I think I will need support from my doctoral coordination or subject matter expert to ensure I analyze that data correctly. I would also like help to review my poster before presenting at the university poster presentation event.

   c. Describe any potential obstacles you anticipate and how your chosen strategies will address them.
   I am not sure I will be through IRB before starting the experience so the timing might change. I am nervous that the parents may not allow me to complete the assessment on their children.

3. Draft a project schedule:

a. Divide your project into major milestones and assign each one a tentative due date and approximate amount of time in the grid below. Include buffer time in your timeline for unforeseen delays or obstacles.
Milestones

    i. Complete IRB: Weeks 1–2: 10 hours?
    ii. Recruit participants: After IRB approval, weeks 2–5: 1 hour per week to put out flyers and track responses
    iii. Collect data: Weeks 4–8–30 minutes per interview. 10 participants – 2 hours and 5 hours planning
    iv. Evaluate data: Weeks 8–10 – looking for themes, 20 hours
    v. Publish or present data: 2 hours and 2 hours to create poster.

b. Evaluate your schedule. Which steps would need support from your mentor? Are there any steps that may require additional time? Are there any overlapping or concurrent steps? Adjust as necessary.

Table 11.3 Project Schedule Example

Week/ insert date	What project objective will be addressed? *There are weeks where there will be no time dedicated to a project objective as you will be at your experience.*	Comments: *How long will this step take? Do you need support from others/mentors to achieve this step?*
Week 1	Complete IRB – week 1–2	2 hours – With PI
Week 2	Complete IRB – week 1–2 Recruit participants	2 hours – With PI 1 hour – with site mentor
Week 3	Recruit participants	1 hour – with site mentor
Week 4	Recruit participants Collect data	1 hour – with site mentor 2 hours – two participants
Week 5	Recruit participants Collect data	1 hour – with site mentor 3 hours – three participants
Week 6	Collect data	3 hours – three participants
Week 7	Collect data	2 hours – two participants
Week 8	Collect data	Buffer time 2 hours – two participants
Week 9	Collect data	Buffer time 2 hours – two participants
Week 10	Evaluate data	5–7 hours with PI
Week 11	Evaluate data Develop poster for dissemination	5–7 hours with PI 1 hour
Week 12	Evaluate data Develop poster for dissemination	Buffer time: 5–7 hours with PI 1 hour
Week 13	Develop poster for dissemination	2 hours + 1 hour buffer
Week 14	Poster presentation data	2 hours + 1 hour buffer

Note: Total hours dedicated to project: 40–45 hours over 14 weeks.

Approved Problem Statement

The problem is a lack of occupation-based evaluation tools utilized to link occupational participation to health, well-being, and quality of life to improve occupational engagement for youth who are overweight/obese and aged 8–16 (Nielsen & Christensen, 2018; Vittrup & McClure, 2018).

Approved Purpose Statement

The purpose of this qualitative research capstone project is to pilot the Pizzi Healthy Weight Management Assessment on youth aged 8–16 to improve health, well-being, quality of life, and occupational engagement for youth who are overweight/obese.

(Roberts – student sample)

References

Nielsen, S. S., & Christensen, J. R. (2018). Occupational Therapy for Adults with Overweight And Obesity: Mapping Interventions Involving Occupational Therapists. *Occupational Therapy International, 2018*.

Vittrup, B., & McClure, D. (2018). Barriers to Childhood Obesity Prevention: Parental Knowledge and Attitudes. *Pediatric Nursing, 44*(2).

Worksheet 11.2: Project Objective Deliverables

Projects produce results of the project activities. These are called deliverables.

Project deliverables can be simple or complex depending on the project activity. The project deliverables can be agreed upon by the doctoral coordinator, student, and mentor(s) so all involved in the project understand when steps are achieved.

In Worksheet 11.1, you identified the steps to your project.

Table 11.4 Project Objectives

List your project objectives:	Briefly plan the objective:	Identify a deliverable for the steps of the project:
1		
2		
3		
4		
5		
6		

List any challenges you can anticipate:

-
-
-
-
-

What strategies can you put into place to overcome or prevent these challenges?

_____

_____

_____

_____

Worksheet 11.2 Example A: Project Objective Deliverables

Program and Policy-Type Project

Projects produce results of the project activities. These are called deliverables.

Project deliverables can be simple or complex depending on the project activity. The project deliverables can be agreed upon by the doctoral coordinator, student, and mentor(s) so all involved in the project understand when steps are achieved.

In Worksheet 11.1, you identified the steps to your project.

Table 11.5 Project Objectives Example A

List your project objectives:	Briefly plan the objective:	Identify a deliverable for the steps of the project:
1. Develop a program.	I will develop four program sessions that will be offered one day per week for four weeks.	Prior to running each session, I will submit the session plan to my mentor for feedback.
2. Implement the program	I am hoping for eight participants per session. I am planning the sessions so that a person can miss one and still participate.	Each week after I offer the program, I can submit a program outline for feedback and review
3. Track progress	I will keep track of what goes well, and what needs improvement at each session.	I will take attendance and collect session feedback forms.
4. Complete a quality enhancement plan	At the end of each session and at the end of all four program sessions, I will collect a participant feedback form.	I can submit the participant feedback forms.
5. Develop a policy for sustainability of the program	After meeting with leadership, I will write a policy and procedure to be given to the site, so the program can continue.	I will submit the policy and procedures in a manual to my mentor.
6		
7		
8		

List any challenges you can anticipate:

I am nervous that I will not be able to get participants for the program.

> **What strategies can you put into place to overcome or prevent these challenges?**
> I can work with my site mentor and capstone team to develop a motivational and fun way to advertise for the program.

Worksheet 11.2 Example B: Project Objective Deliverables

Advocacy-Type Project

Projects produce results of the project activities. These are called deliverables. Project deliverables can be simple or complex depending on the project activity. The project deliverables can be agreed upon by the doctoral coordinator, student, and mentor(s) so all involved in the project understand when steps are achieved.

In Worksheet 11.1, you identified the steps to your project.

Table 11.6 Project Objectives Example B

List your project objectives:	*Briefly plan the objective:*	*Identify a deliverable for the steps of the project:*
1. Identify what you will be advocating and to whom. (For example: community or facility leadership, government officials, social media, civic groups, non-profit leadership or stakeholders relevant to your area of interest.)	I will be advocating for inclusion of occupational therapy services in the transition team for students with severe disabilities at my local high school.	I can submit the name, email and phone number of each point of contact. My plan is to include a representative from: a) school leadership, b) the county school board, c) the occupational therapist(s) at the school, and d) a local non-profit that serves parents of children with severe disabilities.
2. Conduct stakeholder analysis and engagement planning.	I will review the mission of each organization. I need to understand the funding, goals, and current limitations of the current transition program.	I can track and submit what I learn from the analysis on a Google Doc. Then I can meet with each point of contact to review my findings to ensure I am understanding and whether they have any other points of view.
3. Develop a clear message and communication strategy.	I will create documents, brochures, or white papers that identify the current functions and challenges of the transition program.	I can submit the document, brochure, or white paper.

163

4. Implement the outreach plan.	I hope to set up a meeting with the points of contact or their representatives to get together for a one hour meeting to learn how to make a positive change for the transition program at my local school. I will use this meeting to network with my points of contact.	I can submit meeting minutes, tracking any action steps identified.
5. Monitor progress.	I will track any suggestions made at the meeting and monitor progress.	I can submit the action steps from the meeting(s) and support ongoing networking.
6. Develop a sustainability plan for the project.	If there is support, I will create a FB group to expand the reach of the advocacy project. Another option is I will identify the most involved point of contact and share the progress made, and find another leader for the group.	I can show the FB group or the information given to the person who will continue to get the group together.

List Any Challenges You Can Anticipate:

I am not sure I will be able to get four points of contact to network. The parents group is very interested, but the occupational therapists at the school are working on overload, and may not be able to participate.

What Strategies Can You Put in Place to Overcome or Prevent These Challenges?

I can partner with the parent group and expand my search into community occupational therapists or private practice OTs. I can also look at other partnership options, such as local organizations, that provide vocational rehabilitation or independent living options.

References

Cooper, O., Springer, C., & Elleman, B. (2023). Occupational Therapy Services for Transition-Age Youth with Moderate to Severe Disabilities: A Scoping Review. *Research Directs in Therapeutic Sciences*, *2*(1).

Theory Development

Given the limited capstone projects that focus on theory development, we are providing some literature to demonstrate frameworks at different stages of development that support OT practice.

Resources for Those Interested in Theory Development

Chapman, K., Dixon, A., Cocks, K., Ehrlich, C., & Kendall, E. (2022). The Dignity Project Framework: An Extreme Citizen Science Framework in Occupational Therapy and Rehabilitation Research. *Australian Occupational Therapy Journal*, 69(6), 742–752.

Chow, J. K., Pickens, N. D., Fletcher, T., Thompson, M., & Bowyer, P. (2023). 'You've Got to Do Something': Developing Occupational Therapists' Role in End-of-Life Care. *OTJR: Occupational Therapy Journal of Research*, 43(1), 109–118.

Dong, B. (2023). A Systematic Review of the Transforming Leadership Literature and Future Outlook. *Journal of Innovation and Development*, 3(1), 54–58.

Lim, Y. Z. G., Honey, A., & McGrath, M. (2022). The Parenting Occupations and Purposes Conceptual Framework: A Scoping Review of 'Doing' Parenting. *Australian Occupational Therapy Journal*, 69(1), 98–111.

Marshall, C. A., Cooke, A., Gewurtz, R., Barbic, S., Roy, L., Ross, C., . . . & Kirsh, B. (2021). Bridging the Transition from Homelessness: Developing an Occupational Therapy Framework. *Scandinavian Journal of Occupational Therapy*, 1–17.

McKinstry, C., Iacono, T., Kenny, A., Hannon, J., & Knight, K. (2020). Applying a Digital Literacy Framework and Mapping Tool to an Occupational Therapy Curriculum. *Australian Occupational Therapy Journal*, 67(3), 210–217.

Wintle, J., Krupa, T., DeLuca, C., & Cramm, H. (2022). Toward a Conceptual Framework for Occupational Therapist-Teacher Collaborations. *Journal of Occupational Therapy, Schools, & Early Intervention*, 15(2), 148–164.

FREQUENTLY ASKED QUESTIONS

1. **How detailed should my project objectives be when I write them the first time?**

   Developing capstone project objectives is an iterative process. This means that after writing objectives for the first time, it is likely they will change or develop over time. A common example is that the first time you write your objectives, the objectives are what you hope to do. This is in comparison to the final objectives written once you and your DCC and mentor have approved the project and objectives. The objectives change as you learn more about what you will be doing.

   Your project objectives should be as clear and concise as can be. In the beginning, objectives can provide a solid overview but this doesn't need excessive detail. As your project develops, focus on defining what your project aims to achieve, and then the objectives will have more clarity.

2. **How can I create realistic and flexible project objectives and a timeline?**

   The timeline is challenging to develop since when the objectives are written it isn't always clear how long each step might take to complete. While making the plan, start by breaking down your project objectives into smaller tasks and estimate the time you think will be needed for each step. Ask your mentors for feedback on the amount of time needed. Remember to factor in buffer time for unexpected delays. Be realistic about your commitments and available time. Finally, remember, the project objectives and timeline are a plan. Being flexible with your objectives and timeline recognizes you may complete the objectives quicker than planned, or they may take longer. Having a well thought out plan allows for your capstone coordinator and mentors to support you along the capstone process.

REFERENCES

American Occupational Therapy Association (2020). Occupational Therapy Practice Framework: Domain and Process – Fourth Edition. *American Journal of Occupational Therapy*, 74(sup_2), 7412410010. https://doi.org/10.5014/ajot.2020.74S2001.

Huescar Hernandez, E., Moreno-Murcia, J. A., Cid, L., Monteiro, D., & Rodrigues, F. (2020). Passion or Perseverance? The Effect of Perceived Autonomy Support and Grit on Academic Performance in College Students. *International Journal of Environmental Research and Public Health*, *17*(6), 2143.

Morris, T. H. (2020). Experiential Learning – A Systematic Review and Revision of Kolb's Model. *Interactive Learning Environments*, *28*(8), 1064–1077.

Schippers, M. C., Morisano, D., Locke, E. A., Scheepers, A. W., Latham, G. P., & de Jong, E. M. (2020). Writing about Personal Goals and Plans Regardless of Goal Type Boosts Academic Performance. *Contemporary Educational Psychology*, *60*, 101823.

Shorey, S., Chan, V., Rajendran, P., & Ang, E. (2021). Learning Styles, Preferences and Needs Of Generation Z Healthcare Students: Scoping Review. *Nurse Education In Practice*, *57*, 103247.

van Lent, M., & Souverijn, M. (2020). Goal Setting and Raising the Bar: A Field Experiment. *Journal of Behavioral and Experimental Economics*, *87*, 101570.

12

Defending the Planned Project and the Experience

Welcome to this exciting point of your OTD journey. At this point, you have an evidence-based problem, a project planned, and you are getting ready to start the capstone experience. At some point, your academic institution will be verifying that your work meets the expectations of your curriculum.

This chapter will show you examples of what is needed to make sure your project and experience meets the academic standards of your institution. To pass this milestone, you need more than just a rough plan, you need to be able to verbalize or defend what you will be doing for your project and experience. You need to be able to organize yourself and describe to others the value of your project and experience.

> For OTD, instead of a traditional defense, there are checkpoints ensuring project quality, mentor expertise, and comprehensive experience. These checkpoints are described together in this workbook as a defense.

A side note about use of the word defense: Traditionally, the defense for doctoral level work is done at the completion of the project; however, for the entry-level OTD, the student will have checkpoints, so your institution tracks that your project is well-developed, your mentor has verified expertise, and your experience is planned to provide an in-depth experience. You will be defending the plans for your project and alignment of the experience.

Worksheet 12.1 has components required of all academic programs (ACOTE, 2023). Your academic institution may have additional requirements.

Common requirements include:

1. **Literature review**: A literature review grounds the capstone in existing knowledge, identifies gaps or problems, and constructs a framework to frame the capstone project. A comprehensive literature review increases the likelihood that the student understands the context surrounding the project and will have a broader perspective during the experience.
2. **Needs assessment**: The needs assessment identifies specific needs within a population or setting, ensuring that the capstone addresses relevant, real-world issues and increases the likelihood of developing a project that is relevant and impactful.
3. **Goals and objectives**: Clear, measurable goals and objectives for the project and the experience provide direction, purpose, and measurability for the project. Having clear objectives enables structured progression through the project and the experience. Communicating the goals and objectives in writing increases the likelihood that the project's outcomes align with the plan. Having the plan in writing also allows formal and informal mentors to provide support at the appropriate times.

DOI: 10.4324/9781003525868-13

4. **Evaluation plan:** An evaluation plan provides a structured method for measuring project and experiential outcomes, assessing effectiveness and ensuring that the goals and objectives are met. There will be normative and summative types of evaluation throughout the time of your capstone project and experience. There is likely going to be a list of 'things' that the student will provide to demonstrate progress over the 14 weeks. These 'things' are variable based on a student project and are referred to in this workbook as deliverables.

5. **Experiential plan, affiliation agreement, contract, or memorandum of understanding (MOU):** The experiential plan formalizes a site, setting, or facility to the academic institution. The experiential plan demonstrates collaboration between the student, academic institution, and a site by outlining specific capstone objectives; plans for evaluation and mentoring; and responsibilities of the institution, student, and site. Having a signed document allows for discussions between all involved to increase clarity, accountability, and increases the likelihood of uninterrupted progression of the project. Before beginning the experience, the student, academic program, and site agree on objectives you will meet at the site. These objectives are in addition to your project, and will contribute to the site. A plan to evaluate your progress towards the experience/site objectives are generally included in the MOU.

6. **Mentor agreement (optional):** The mentor agreement is variable depending on the academic institution and the category of mentors that can be utilized. Academic institutions determine the mentor type for students to enhance the capstone project and experience. At a minimum, the project is mentored by faculty and a content mentor (or subject matter expert, SME). Then the experience is developed with specific plans for evaluation and mentoring. Before beginning the project, the student, academic program, and mentor agree on objectives you will meet for your capstone (project and/or experience). A plan to evaluate your progress towards the objectives is generally included in the mentor agreement. The mentor agreement can be a written agreement between the academic institution and the mentor, or there may be assigned faculty to mentor the capstone experience. For programs that allow mentorship from individuals outside of the academic setting, there may be a written mentor agreement. A written mentor agreement is a signed document similar to the contract or memorandum of understanding (MOU). The mentor agreement serves to verify that the student receives mentorship during the capstone experience. The person serving as the mentor must have documented or verified expertise in an aspect of the student's area of interest.

By the end of this chapter, you will be able to effectively defend your capstone project and meet all of your academic institution's many requirements.

The defense serves as a checkpoint to verify that each student can effectively 'make their case' and has:

- Developed a capstone project that meets the academic program's expectations,
- Planned a capstone experience that provides concentration in the designated area of interest.

The defense increases the likelihood that once the planned project and experience are complete, the student will successfully demonstrate a synthesis and application of knowledge in their chosen area of interest.

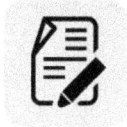

Worksheet 12.1: Meeting the Requirements

Prior to starting the capstone experience, each student will demonstrate the requirements listed in the far left column of Table 12.1.

Use this worksheet to demonstrate how you can plan to show you have met the requirements.

Your academic institution may provide you with more requirements, or provide specific strategies to show these requirements have been met. This worksheet serves as a guide.

Table 12.1 Meeting the Requirements

Requirement	Met by (Options)	Circle one		Comments/ reflection. What is the next step to complete this requirement?
Literature review	A completed literature review Chapter 2	Met	Not Met	
Needs assessment	Conceptual framework SWOT SOAR PESTLE Normative need Comparative need Component of Chapter 3	Met	Not Met	
Goals/objectives	Learning (experiential/ site) objectives Project objectives Time log Component of Chapter 3	Met Met Met	Not Met Not Met Not Met	
Evaluation plan	Learning (experiential/ site) objectives – How will they be measured Project objectives – How will they be measured? Time log – How will time be tracked? Component of Chapter 3	Met Met Met	Not Met Not Met Not Met	
Memorandum of understanding (MOU or contract)	Completed MOU	Met	Not Met	
Mentored practice setting or experiential requirements	Background check Drug screen CPR Vaccinations	Met Met Met Met	Not Met Not Met Not Met Not Met	

Requirement	Met by (Options)	Circle one		Comments/ reflection. What is the next step to complete this requirement?
Mentor agreement Mentored by an individual with expertise	Signed mentor form (one form per mentor) Documentation of mentor expertise (Mentor CV/resume)	Met Met	Not Met Not Met	

Worksheet 12.2: Draft a Presentation that Supports the Capstone Project and Experience

1. What is the title of your project?
2. Background

   a. Briefly summarize research literature related to the scope of the study topic
   b. Describe the gap in knowledge in the discipline that the study will address and why the study is needed
   c. Describe how the problem, purpose, and experience relate to occupation and occupational therapy.

3. Problem Statement

   a. State the problem
   b. Provide evidence of consensus that the problem is current, relevant, and significant to the discipline
   c. Frame the problem in a way that builds upon or counters previous research findings focusing on the problem
   d. Address a meaningful gap in the current research literature
   e. Ensure the problem is directly related to occupational therapy.

4. Purpose of the Project

   a. State the purpose
   b. Indicate the project type
   c. Defend the purpose and project type from the literature
   d. State the variables and/or concept/phenomenon (as appropriate to the particular study)
   e. Based on the needs assessment, and collaboration with you mentor and site, defend the purpose and project type.

5. Project Objective or Research Questions

   a. State the research questions or project objectives
   b. For each objective, what is the deliverable to ensure the objective is met?

6. Hypotheses

   a. For research projects – state hypotheses
   b. For all other project types – from the project you have planned, what are your desired outcomes and deliverables?

c. Defend that the hypotheses, outcomes, and deliverables are linked to the profession.

7. Conceptual or Theoretical Framework

a. Name of theory, frame of reference, or model
b. Identify author of the theory
c. State how your project is planned or framed by the theory and how the theory interfaces with your project.

8. Method/Design/Process and Method

a. Describe what you will be doing for your project
b. Ensure each objective was met with a deliverable (aka what others can evaluate)
c. What is the time requirement for each objective and deliverable?
d. For each objective, answer 'Using this (method/process) will allow me to . . .'

9. Data/Information Collection Technique

a. How will you track action towards objectives?
b. How will you ensure you are meeting your objectives?

10. Impact Statement

a. Describe potential implications for positive social and occupational change that can occur from the project
b. Describe the plan for sustainability of the project.

11. Mentor/Site Communication and Support

a. What will be done when you have an in-depth (14-week) experience? Briefly describe learning (experiential) objectives as applicable
b. Describe your site and identify site mentors
c. What support and guidance will be needed to ensure your project is successful?
d. How will the support and guidance be provided by the mentor, site mentor, or other stakeholders?

12. Concluding Thoughts

a. Provide a strong 'take home' message that captures the key essence of the project.

13. Acknowledgements

a. Thank your committee members
b. Thank the doctoral coordinators
c. Thank your classmates
d. Thank family and friends.

14. References

FREQUENTLY ASKED QUESTIONS

1. **What is the most important objective of capstone plan defense?** The main purpose of the capstone plan defense is to demonstrate your understanding of your area of interest, your ability to describe your capstone project, and your capstone experience. This way, your academic institution, mentor, and capstone experience site can better support the completion of the project, and suggest relevant opportunities available during the experience.

2. **What presentation format should I anticipate for the capstone plan defense?** Since the defense is variable per academic institution, there is no specific format. It may be as simple as checkpoints to make sure each of the requirements are complete, or a formal presentation to faculty and peers. If there is a capstone plan defense presentation, it consists of a formal PowerPoint, Canva, or other slide-based presentation of your project, followed by a Q&A session with the committee members.

3. **How long should my capstone plan defense presentation be?** Depending on the institution, a defense presentation typically lasts between 15 and 45 minutes.

4. **During the defense, what sorts of questions will committee members and participants ask?** People who take the time to attend your defense will be interested in making sure you have the best project and experience possible. The worksheet plan in this chapter aims to address the most common questions by including them in the presentation.

   a. Can you briefly summarize your research or project?
   b. What motivated or inspired you to select this topic/research question in particular?
   c. What contribution does your project make to the profession of occupational therapy?
   d. What contribution does your experience make to the population or profession of occupational therapy?
   e. What were the most difficult obstacles you encountered in your research, and how did you overcome them?
   f. How did you choose your project type, and why did you believe it was the best fit for your capstone problem?
   g. What implications does your research have for the profession of occupational therapy or area of interest?
   h. If you were speaking to a group of stakeholders, what is the significance of your project?
   i. What is the one thing you would like us to remember about your capstone project?

5. **How should I prepare for possible questions or feedback?** Review the development of your project in detail and anticipate potential questions. If possible, give practice or mock defenses with peers or mentors, and see the types of questions participants have. Although you should be prepared to 'defend' your choices, be receptive to constructive criticism or feedback. Your faculty, your mentors, and your doctoral capstone coordinator want you to have the best possible project and experience. Feedback is there to help you make changes before the project or experience begins.

REFERENCES

Accreditation Council for Occupational Therapy Education (ACOTE) (2023). 2023 Accreditation Council for Occupational Therapy Education (ACOTE®) Standards and Interpretive Guide. Retrieved from: https://acoteonline.org/accreditation-explained/standards/.

American Occupational Therapy Association (2020). Occupational Therapy Practice Framework: Domain and Process – Fourth Edition. *American Journal of Occupational Therapy*, *74*(sup_2), 7412410010. https://doi.org/10.5014/ajot.2020.74S2001.

Fleming, R. S., & Kowalsky, M. (2021). *Survival Skills for Thesis and Dissertation Candidates*. Springer.

Ho, Y. R., Chen, B. Y., & Li, C. M. (2023). Thinking More Wisely: Using the Socratic Method to Develop Critical Thinking Skills Amongst Healthcare Students. *BMC Medical Education*, *23*(1), 173.

13

Planning and Tracking the Experience

As you start your doctoral capstone experience, it's important to plan for the experience, and keep track of your specific objectives, supervision, and mentorship. Your capstone experience gives you the opportunity to apply your knowledge, skills, and abilities in the real world. Making best use of this time benefits you and your population of interest.

For example, if you are planning a program and policy development-type capstone project, but also want to practice advocacy and leadership skills, you will need to make a plan with a schedule of when you will meet the project objectives and the experience objectives. Writing the plan the first time can be challenging since you won't be perfectly clear about everything you can accomplish during your experience. There is flexibility in the plan, and your site, mentor, and DCC understand there will be changes.

Table 13.1 Examples for Capstone Project Objectives

Clinical Practice Skills	1. Get approvals for the plan of specific clinical practice skill(s) to be implemented 2. Recruit clients or relevant individuals 3. Track provision of clinical practice skills in alignment with the plan 4. Monitor the outcomes 5. Complete quality assurance measures with clients and supervisors or mentors 6. Publish or present a clinical pathway describing the guidelines for best practice implementation of the clinical practice skill(s).
Research Type	1. Complete IRB (ideally, before the start of the experience). 2. Recruit participants 3. Collect data 4. Evaluate data 5. Publish or present data.
Administration	There are common threads in project types between administration and leadership. For these examples, administration is at a group or departmental level. Get approvals for the planned objective type. For example: Workflow metrics, staff training system development, resource allocation, burnout prevention 1. Implement the planned objective 2. Track progress 3. Complete a quality assurance plan 4. Publish or present on the project outcomes.

(Continued)

DOI: 10.4324/9781003525868-14

Table 13.1 (Continued)

Leadership	There are common threads in project types between administration and leadership. For these examples, leadership is at an organizational level. 1. Disseminate the planned objective type. For example: Strategic growth planning; diversity, equity and inclusion initiatives; conflict resolution; analysis of legal, fiscal, or regulatory factors; organizational effectiveness initiatives 2. Implement the planned objective 3. Track progress 4. Complete a quality assurance plan 5. Publish or present on the project outcomes.
Program and Policy Development	1. Develop a program (ideally, this is started before the start of the experience) 2. Implement the program 3. Track progress 4. Complete a quality enhancement plan 5. Develop a policy for sustainability for the program 6. Publish or present on the program and policy outcomes.
Advocacy	1. Identify what you will be advocating and to whom. For example, community or facility leadership, government officials, social media, civic groups, non-profit leadership, or stakeholders relevant to your area of interest 2. Conduct stakeholder analysis and engagement planning 3. Develop a clear message and communication strategy 4. Implement the outreach plan. 5. Monitor progress 6. Develop a sustainability plan for the project 7. Publish or present on the advocacy outcomes.
Education	1. Identify the gap in knowledge for a specific population/audience 2. Design the curriculum, objectives, and course outlines 3. Develop the educational modules, training sessions, or continuing education units (CEU) 4. Schedule the education session(s) 5. Track participant progress 6. Develop a sustainability plan for the educational module(s) 7. Publish or present on the educational outcomes.
Theory Development	Note: Theory development can overlap with all other project types. 1. Determine the stage of development or need for advancement for a particular framework, model, or theory, or determine the need to apply a known framework, model, or theory to a new population. 2. Identify and collaborate with authors, mentors, and scholars who have made notable contributions to the framework, model, or theory. 3. Devise a strategy either to enhance the framework, model, or theory or to implement it specifically for a target population. 4. Develop a sustainability plan for continued development of the framework, theory, or model. 5. Present or publish new hypotheses, redefining concepts, suggesting new relationships, or emphasizing potential applications to the target population and/or authors, mentors, and scholars.

Given the limited capstone projects that focus on theory development, it has been removed as an option from the updated ACOTE standards. However, given the importance of developing profession theories, we are providing some literature to demonstrate frameworks at different stages of development that support OT practice.

Resources for Those Interested in Theory Development:

Chapman, K., Dixon, A., Cocks, K., Ehrlich, C., & Kendall, E. (2022). The Dignity Project Framework: An Extreme Citizen Science Framework in Occupational Therapy and Rehabilitation Research. *Australian Occupational Therapy Journal, 69*(6), 742–752.

Chow, J. K., Pickens, N. D., Fletcher, T., Thompson, M., & Bowyer, P. (2023). 'You've Got to Do Something': Developing Occupational Therapists' Role in End-of-Life Care. *OTJR: Occupational Therapy Journal of Research, 43*(1), 109–118.

Dong, B. (2023). A Systematic Review of the Transforming Leadership Literature and Future Outlook. *Journal of Innovation and Development, 3*(1), 54–58.

Lim, Y. Z. G., Honey, A., & McGrath, M. (2022). The Parenting Occupations and Purposes Conceptual Framework: A Scoping Review of 'Doing' Parenting. *Australian Occupational Therapy Journal, 69*(1), 98–111.

Marshall, C. A., Cooke, A., Gewurtz, R., Barbic, S., Roy, L., Ross, C., . . . & Kirsh, B. (2021). Bridging the Transition from Homelessness: Developing an Occupational Therapy Framework. *Scandinavian Journal of Occupational Therapy*, 1–17.

McKinstry, C., Iacono, T., Kenny, A., Hannon, J., & Knight, K. (2020). Applying a Digital Literacy Framework and Mapping Tool to an Occupational Therapy Curriculum. *Australian Occupational Therapy Journal, 67*(3), 210–217.

Wintle, J., Krupa, T., DeLuca, C., & Cramm, H. (2022). Toward a Conceptual Framework for Occupational Therapist-Teacher Collaborations. *Journal of Occupational Therapy, Schools, & Early Intervention, 15*(2), 148–164.

Once you've started planning your project objectives, start drafting a detailed plan that lists the goals and activities for the project and experience over the 14-week capstone experience. This will help you keep track of your weekly goals. The plan will enable your mentor and site supervisor to coordinate and offer you appropriate support over the course of the experience.

This plan should be made with the help of your DCC, mentor, and/or site supervisor, and it should be looked over and changed as needed to make sure you are on the right track and making progress toward your goals. Keep track of how far you've come and write down any problems or setbacks you face along the way. Your weekly goals will show how your responsibilities are growing at your site.

Use the following samples and worksheet to plan objectives for the capstone project and experience.

Table 13.2 Planning/Estimating for Hours and Weeks to Be Met: Clinical Practice Skills as an Example

1. Get approvals for the plan of specific clinical practice skill(s) to be implemented	2 hours, completed before start date or week 1
2. Recruit clients or relevant individuals	2 hours, week 1–3
3. Track provision of clinical practice skills in alignment with the plan	4 hours per week, week 4–8

4. Monitor the outcomes	1 hour per week, week 4–9
5. Complete quality assurance measures with clients and supervisors or mentors	2 hours, week 8–9
6. Publish or present a clinical pathway describing the guidelines for best practice implementation of the clinical practice skill(s).	2 hours, week 9–10 to put into writing; 2 hours, week 14.

Table 13.3 Examples for Capstone Experience/Site Objectives and Estimated Time Involved

In collaboration with the mentored practice setting, the student will:	
Clinical Practice Skills	*Participate in provision of clinical practice skills. Note: There should be a distinction between these clinical practice skills and a level II fieldwork experience. For example, in addition to evaluation, intervention, and discharge, the student will:*
Research Type	Participate in ongoing research being conducted
Administration	Participate in administration meetings as permitted
Leadership	Participate in leadership and board meetings as permitted
Program and Policy Development	Participate in developing, implementing, or reviewing policies for new or existing programs
Advocacy	Participate in the development, implementation, or evaluation of advocacy efforts
Education	Participate in the development, implementation, or evaluation of educational offerings
Theory Development	Participate in the development, implementation, or evaluation of applicable frameworks, models, or theories.

Table 13.4 Sample Capstone Experience Objectives Timeline, Planning for Hours and Weeks to be Met

Considerations for each category:	
Clinical Skills	*10 hours per week with the interdisciplinary team*
Research	10 hours per week with the research team, 1 hour with the principal investigators, 2 hours with the statistician, 7 hours with the sub-instigator
Administration	4 hours every 3 weeks. Attend the administration meetings
Leadership	4 hours over the 14-week experience
Program and Policy Development	30 hours per week, rotating through the different programs offered
Advocacy	2 hours per week with partner organization
Education	4 hours every month. Participate in the staff training
Theory Development	1 hour per week, progress implementation and evaluation of use of [student chosen's] framework, model, or theory in the department.

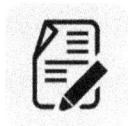

Worksheet 13.1: Capstone Experience Plan

Write your objectives and begin developing your experiential plan.

Individual Capstone Project Objectives (POs):

Note: Using program and policy-type capstone project.

PO1.

PO2.

PO3.

PO4.

PO5.

Individual 14-Week Capstone Experience Objectives (EOs):

In collaboration with the mentored practice setting, the student will:

EO1.

EO2.

EO3.

EO4.

EO5.

Table 13.5 Weekly Schedule/Plan

Weekly Schedule/ Plan: Minimum 14 weeks. Can be longer	Hours	Objectives: Identify which objective	Activities (with specificity)
Week 1			
Total	40		
			Deliverable:
Week 2			
Total	40		

Weekly Schedule/ Plan: Minimum 14 weeks. Can be longer	Hours	Objectives: Identify which objective	Activities (with specificity)
			Deliverable:
Week 3			
Total	40		
			Deliverable:
Week 4			
Total	40		
			Deliverable:

Worksheet 13.1 Example: Capstone Experience Plan

Write your objectives and begin developing your experiential plan.

Individual Capstone Project Objectives (POs):

Note: Using program and policy-type capstone project.

PO1. Develop a program. (Encouraged this is started before the start of the experience).
PO2. Implement the program.
PO3. Track progress.
PO4. Complete a quality enhancement plan.
PO5. Develop a policy for sustainability for the program.
PO6. Publish or present on the program and policy outcomes.

Individual 14-Week Capstone Experience Objectives (EOs):

In collaboration with the mentored practice setting, the student will:

EO1. Engage in administrative or leadership roles and tasks, such as organizing team projects, leading group discussions, or participating in community initiatives.
EO2. The student will understand and contribute to existing programs and services. This participation will include reviewing and applying the established

policies and procedures used for the effective execution of these programs and services.

EO3. Describe OT's potential roles, responsibilities, and funding within the mentored practice setting. (Potential deliverable: Create a job description).

EO4. The student will understand and contribute to existing advocacy efforts. This participation will include reviewing and understanding the advocacy effort at the mentored practice setting and community stakeholders.

EO5. The student will understand and contribute to existing education and training efforts. This participation will include reviewing and understanding the existing educational and training offerings at the mentored practice setting.

Table 13.6 Example of Planned Capstone Experience Time Log

Weekly Schedule/Plan: Minimum 14 weeks. Can be longer	Hours	Objectives: Identify which objective	Activities (with specificity)
Week 1	2	PO1	Conduct a secondary needs assessment to learn types of services provided in comparison to the planned program.
	30	EO2	Orient at the site to meet the leaders, staff, and clients. Develop an understanding of the different functions at the mentored practice setting. Identify where collaboration is best planned.
	5	EO1	Meet with site mentor to review current status of program development. Identify who will be supporting the scheduling and recruitment.
	3	EO2	Complete onboarding and orientation requirements.
Total	40		
			Sample deliverables (to DCC or site supervisor): a. Draft of program plan b. Compare and contrast chart between the population at the mentored practice setting and the population identified in the literature review.
Week 2	5	PO1 and PO2	Based on the secondary needs assessment, complete the development of the first two program modules and present them to the site mentor for feedback. Plan recruitment and schedule for the program.
	5	EO1	In collaboration with the site mentor, seek out the administration or leadership to identify any opportunities to learn about the functions that will occur over the capstone experience time. Schedule and plan participation in administrative or leadership activities.

Weekly Schedule/Plan: Minimum 14 weeks. Can be longer	Hours	Objectives: Identify which objective	Activities (with specificity)
	30	EO2	Collaborate with leaders, staff, or clients identified in week 1 to observe or contribute to existing programs and services. This includes reviewing policy and procedures used in the development and implementation of the programs and services.
Total	40		
			Sample deliverables (to DCC or site supervisor): a. Draft of modified program plan. b. Compare and contrast chart between the services and professionals at the mentored practice setting and the services identified in the literature review.
Week 3	30	EO2	Contribute to existing programs and services. This includes reviewing policy and procedures used in the development and implementation of the programs and services. Gain knowledge and experience from program leaders and advice on how to work with the population.
	5	PO1 and PO2	Finalize the occupation-based program with site supervisor and project mentor, to begin week 4. Includes scheduling and recruitment.
	5	No linked objective – indirect hours	The student will participate in a 5-hour continuing education class related to their capstone.
Total	40		
			Sample deliverables (to DCC or site supervisor): a. Course completion document from CE course. b. Student will write a reflection paper detailing their comprehension of the policies and procedures associated with the existing programs and services.
Week 4	4	PO2 and PO3	Start planned program. 2 hours per session, 2 days per week.
	30	EO2	Contribute to existing programs and services with increasing participation in collaboration with mentored practice setting.
	1	PO3 and PO4	Meet with site mentor to get feedback of program sessions.

Weekly Schedule/Plan: Minimum 14 weeks. Can be longer	Hours	Objectives: Identify which objective	Activities (with specificity)
	5	EO4 May be off mentored practice setting	Collaborate with leaders, staff, or clients identified in week 1 to observe or contribute to advocacy efforts. This may include going to an established community partnership.
Total	40		
			Deliverable: The student will provide a reflection or summary highlighting the strengths and weaknesses observed during the program sessions of the first week. The student will summarize the current status of advocacy efforts at the mentored practice setting.

Worksheet 13.2: Weekly Evaluation of Experiential Plan

Purpose: Use this form to document your hours and progress towards your experiential plan.

Student Name:
Date:
Number of week/total weeks: Week # _____ Expected weeks to complete # _____ (Minimum is 14 weeks)
Hours completed this week: _____

Table 13.7 Experimental Plan Hours and Progress Form

Site(s) name

(Identify site and dates of experiential time for project and experience per site, and indicate who will be approved to sign the experiential weekly time log and objective form)

Site 1: _____   Days: M T W T F
Person approving form: _____
Site 2: _____   Days: M T W T F
Person approving form: _____
(Add as needed)

Learning objectives: Write all experience or learning objectives addressed this week here (i.e., objectives that have been developed related to your capstone and that are not directly related to the project type).

Identify the learning objectives you worked on this week from your time log:

EO1.

EO2.

Project objectives: Write all project objectives addressed this week here (i.e., objectives developed for the project type).

Identify the project objectives you worked on this week from your time log:

PO1.

PO2.

Weekly sched-ule/plan: What was planned?	Hours spent per activity:	Activities (with specificity):	Time with mentor over the week:	Objective met or not met with comment:

Mentor Signature: _____Date: _____

or/and

Site Supervisor: _____ **Date**: _____

Worksheet 13.3: Experiential Plan Deliverables Submission

Student Name:
 Date:
 Number of week/Total Weeks: Week # _____ Expected weeks to complete #

Table 13.8 Weekly Evaluation of Experiential Plan

Learning/experiential objectives – Write all learning objectives addressed this week here (These are directly from your time log document. If an additional objective was met this week, indicate the change/addition)
EO
EO
EO
Project Objectives – Write all project objectives addressed this week here (Objectives developed for the project type)
PO
PO
Deliverable – Submit deliverable here or as an attached document (Objectives developed for the project type)
Per the time log: (Or see attached/ additional document)

FREQUENTLY ASKED QUESTIONS

1. **What is the difference when planning the capstone project versus the capstone experience?**

   The capstone experience is an immersive opportunity designed to give the student the opportunity to develop a deeper understanding of the 'area of interest.' The experience can be at different locations and provides varied access points supporting the area of interest. For example, the experience could include participating at an organization and performing tasks from any project type.

   In contrast, the capstone project entails completion of the capstone project, which was developed and approved. For example, if the approved project was a program and policy-type project, there will be specific deliverables of a program and policy to demonstrate the project was completed.

2. **What is the best way to divide my time between the project and the capstone experience?**

   There is no best way. Creating a timeline, and planning how much time will be spent on the project versus the experience is one way to develop your professional skills. Time allocation varies based on the amount of time needed to develop the project. For example, a program and policy-type project may require 4 hours per week, for 6 weeks, weeks 3–8 (total of 24 on-site hours for the project). Around those weeks, the experience time will include these hours. On the other hand, a quantitative research-type capstone may only require 4 hours for data analysis, week 10 (total of 4 off-site hours).

It is advisable to balance your schedule with adequate (full-time) immersion at the capstone experience site, and then layer in your capstone project obligations.

3. **Can the capstone experience and capstone project hours overlap?**

Yes, the project and experience hours may, in fact, overlap. They don't have to, but they can. Students can plan a capstone project and find a site where the project hours are done on-site for the capstone experience. On the other hand, a student might complete a project outside of a capstone experience site, and the hours will not contribute to the experiential hours.

4. **How can I effectively manage my time throughout the capstone experience phase?**

Developing effective time management skills requires establishing specific objectives, breaking the objectives into smaller tasks, prioritizing the tasks, and writing the steps into a timeline. Seeking mentor feedback and evaluating your progress allows you to develop your time management skills.

REFERENCES

American Occupational Therapy Association (2020). Occupational Therapy Practice Framework: Domain and Process – Fourth Edition. *American Journal of Occupational Therapy*, *74*(sup_2), 7412410010. https://doi.org/10.5014/ajot.2020.74S2001.

Huescar Hernandez, E., Moreno-Murcia, J. A., Cid, L., Monteiro, D., & Rodrigues, F. (2020). Passion or Perseverance? The Effect of Perceived Autonomy Support and Grit on Academic Performance in College Students. *International Journal of Environmental Research and Public Health*, *17*(6), 2143.

Morris, T. H. (2020). Experiential Learning – A Systematic Review and Revision of Kolb's Model. *Interactive Learning Environments*, *28*(8), 1064–1077.

Schippers, M. C., Morisano, D., Locke, E. A., Scheepers, A. W., Latham, G. P., & de Jong, E. M. (2020). Writing about Personal Goals and Plans Regardless of Goal Type Boosts Academic Performance. *Contemporary Educational Psychology*, *60*, 101823.

Shorey, S., Chan, V., Rajendran, P., & Ang, E. (2021). Learning Styles, Preferences and Needs Of Generation Z Healthcare Students: Scoping Review. *Nurse Education In Practice*, *57*, 103247.

Tarasova, E. N., Khatsrinova, O., Fakhretdinova, G. N., & Kaybiyaynen, A. A. (2021). Project-based Learning Activities for Engineering College Students. In *Educating Engineers for Future Industrial Revolutions: Proceedings of the 23rd International Conference on Interactive Collaborative Learning (ICL2020)*, Volume 2 (pp. 253–260). Springer International Publishing.

van Lent, M., & Souverijn, M. (2020). Goal Setting and Raising the Bar: A Field Experiment. *Journal of Behavioral and Experimental Economics*, *87*, 101570.

14

Unveiling Your Outcomes: The Capstone Project Outcomes

THE RESULTS, THE FINDINGS, THE OUTCOMES OFTEN SYNONYMOUS WITH 'CHAPTER 4'

You have completed an individual capstone project to showcase your ability to synthesize and apply what you have learned about your area of interest. It's time to bring everything you've learned and share the outcomes of you project.

How will you share your outcomes? This varies between academic institutions. This chapter describes information your institution might ask about in regards to project outcomes.

You will describe the outcomes of your capstone project in this section. For the purposes of the workbook, we will refer to this section as Chapter 4. Chapter 4 is when you revisit the project objectives identified in Chapter 3 and systematically organize and describe what happened during the implementation of the project. This section, or Chapter 4, focuses only on the project's objectives. Do not include any of your opinions, just describe factually what happened as your project was implemented and completed.

Menu

- **Introduction**: Restate the original problem, purpose, rationale, and significance that provided the foundation for the project.
- **Restate the project objectives:** This section is included to restate and clarify the project objectives, ensuring the objectives align with the presented findings.
- **Describe the setting:** Detail the setting to provide context, allowing the reader to understand the environment in which the project took place and that influenced the project. For research projects this might be where you recruited participants.
- **Time frame:** Describing duration or time frame offers insight into the scope and potential limitations of the project.
- **Participants/stakeholders:** This section describes the demographics, relevant characteristics, or sample size of the people who participated in the project. Provide a clear picture of who was involved in the project.
- **Development/design:** This section highlights the evolution and progression of the project process, offering a behind-the-scenes look at how the project unfolded. This includes phases and/or changes made along the capstone journey.
- **Evaluation/analysis:** An evaluation or analysis allows for a critical assessment of the implemented strategies, data analysis, or the effectiveness of the project. The reader understands how the data or strategies were processed and interpreted.

DOI: 10.4324/9781003525868-15

- **Results/findings:** Present the findings, offering the tangible outcomes of the capstone project. Allow the reader to draw inferences and understand the implications of the project.
- **Conclusion:** Summarizing the entirety of the project. The conclusion ties together all aspects of the project process and outcomes.

Table 14.1 Sample Content to Detail Project Outcomes

Written factually and in comparison to the individual project objectives:

Program and Policy-Type Project	Research-Type Project	Leadership-Type Project
Objectives: Restate the project objectives	Objectives: Restate the project objectives	Objectives: Restate the project objectives
Setting: Describe where the program was implemented	Setting: Describe where participants were recruited	Setting: Describe the organization(s) where the project was implemented
Time frame: Over what duration was the program implemented?	Time frame: Over what duration was the research collected?	Time frame: Over what duration was the leadership project implemented?
Participants: Describe characteristics of the participants	Participants: Describe characteristics of the participants, inclusion/exclusion criteria, report demographic data	Participants: Describe characteristics of the context, people, leaders, or stakeholders involved
Development: Based on the literature and needs assessment, describe how the program session(s) were developed and why this was needed	Development: Based on the literature and needs assessment, state the research questions and hypotheses	Development: Based on the literature and needs assessment, describe how the leadership project was developed and why it was needed
Program evaluation: Describe how the outcomes of the program were measured	Design: Describe the research design	Leadership blueprint, audit or roadmap: Describe how the outcomes of the leadership project were measured
Analysis: Analyze the outcomes of the program.	Analysis: Analyze the data collected.	Analysis: Analyze the outcomes of the leadership project
Results: Report participant satisfaction, tables, figures, or charts that share the key outcomes of the program	Results: Report data, tables, figures, or charts that share the key outcomes of the program	Results: Report performance indicators, participant satisfaction, tables, figures, or charts that share the key outcomes of the program
Conclusion: Summarize the outcomes of the project. State broadly how the objectives were met or not met and directly contributed to solve the problem	Conclusion: Summarize the outcomes of the project. State broadly how the objectives were met or not met and how they directly contributed to solve the problem	Conclusion: Summarize the outcomes of the project. State broadly how the objectives were met or not met and directly contributed to solve the problem

EXAMPLE 1

Each section of the capstone writing should be self-contained. What this means is that a reader should be able to pick up any section of your writing and have an understanding of the project and objectives without having to refer to previous writing.

Template

The purpose of this chapter is to provide an overview of the results of the capstone project. This chapter will report on the outcomes of the project related to the problem of XYZ (restate problem). The purpose of this project was to (restate purpose). (Restate research questions as applicable). The project occurred over (insert dates). The goal of reporting the outcomes and providing an analysis is to compare the findings as related to the literature review and report the outcomes to evidence synthesis of the knowledge of the (insert area/population of interest) and application of the knowledge.

Sample

The purpose of this chapter is to provide an overview of the results of the capstone project. This chapter will report on the outcomes of the project related to the problem of insufficient mental health services for formerly incarcerated women, which negatively impacts their life skills for community reintegration (Dillon et al., 2020; Jaegers et al., 2020; Salem et al., 2021). The purpose of this program development-type capstone project was to create, implement, and evaluate a mental health occupational therapy program for formerly incarcerated women re-integrating into the community. The project occurred from _____ to _____. The goal of reporting the outcomes and providing an analysis is to compare the findings as related to the literature review and report the outcomes to evidence synthesis of the knowledge of incarcerated women who are reintegrating back into the community and application of the knowledge (Viles, 2024 – student sample).

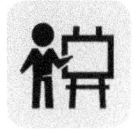

Learning Activity 14.1: Introduction

Your introduction should serve as a brief overview that revisits the main reasons behind your project.

The Original Problem:

What was the problem you aimed to address with your project? Problem statement:

_____

_____

The Original Purpose or Project Type:

What was the purpose of your project, and what was the project type? Purpose statement:

_____

_____

Draft Your Introductory Paragraph (Refer to Sample in Learning Activity 1):

S1: The purpose of this chapter is to provide an overview of the results of the capstone project (main idea).

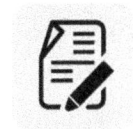

S2: This chapter will report on the outcomes of the project related to the problem.

(Citations: Citation 1_____, Citation 2_____)
S3: The purpose of this _____-type capstone project was to create, implement, and evaluate.

S4: The project occurred from

S5: The goal of reporting the outcomes and providing an analysis is to compare the findings as related to the literature review and report the outcomes to evidence synthesis of the knowledge of

---

EXAMPLE 2

This is an example that details the following:

Setting, Time Frame, Participants or Stakeholders, and Project Design

Setting:

Program and policy-type project: The program was discussed with _____ and _____. Once the program was approved, an attempt was made to seek program approval from _____. However, the deadline for program approval had passed. The program was then marketed to _____ and was approved to be implemented as part of the project (Viles, 2023 – student sample).

   Research-type project: Participants were recruited from virtual platforms including: _____

Time Frame:

The program ran for the planned duration of 5 weeks, face-to-face, 3 hours per week without any changes.

Participants:

The original inclusion and exclusion participant criteria had to be modified to fit the experiential site's criteria. The original participants were planned to be male or female participants. Due to the site, participants were women between the ages of 18 and 65 who have been justice-impacted (incarceration in jail/prison or community control) at any time in their lives and need assistance with reentry. Participants could only participate in the program post-incarceration because that was the mission of the organization.

Project Design (including changes from original plan):

A secondary needs assessment was conducted on-site, and a pre-survey was administered to collect information on the needs of the participants. The information gathered was used to guide the development of the program sessions and activities. Each week a new topic was presented. The overall goal of the program was to provide the participants with coping strategies, practical skills, and the development of healthy habits to overcome challenges they may face upon community reentry.

Each session was focused on a stand-alone topic, not scaffolding upon previous sessions. The program was conducted this way due to the scheduling differences and difficulties of the participants. Cole's Seven-Step Groups format was used to guide the structure of each session: introduction, activity, sharing, processing, generalizing, application, and summary (Cole, 2017). The five topics include: social participation, stress management, goal setting and goal achievement, roles, and health exploration. Each week the participants engaged in self-reflection activities and group sharing.

Learning Activity 14.2: Setting, Time Frame, Participants or Stakeholders, and Development Design

1. Original planned setting or recruitment sources:

   _____

   _____

2. Were there any changes in setting? If yes, what was the change?

   _____

   _____

3. What details can you provide about your context or setting that influenced your project?

   _____

   _____

4. What was the time frame of your planned project? (How many months, days, or hours?)

   _____

   _____

5. Were there any changes made between your planned project time frame and the actual time frame of the project? If yes, what was the change?

_____

_____

6. What details can you provide about the time frame that relates to the scope or limitations of the project?

_____

_____

7. Who were the original participants or stakeholders (or organizations) targeted for your planned project?

_____

_____

8. Were there any changes from the original participants or stakeholders from the plan to the actual project?

_____

_____

9. What details can you provide about the participants or stakeholders that relates to the scope or limitations of the project?

_____

_____

Briefly describe the original project plan.

10. Were there any differences between the original project plan and the actual implementation of the project?

_____

_____

11. What details can you provide about the original plan compared to the actual project that relate to the scope, limitations, or assumptions of the project?

_____

_____

Using Example 2 and the information written in Learning Activity 14.2, draft your sections for the setting, time frame, participants or stakeholders, and development design:

State the information about the setting of your project:

_____

_____

State the time frame of your project:

_____

_____

State the participants or stakeholders:

_____

_____

State the project design:

_____

_____

EXAMPLE 3

This is an example that details the following: Evaluation and analysis, results/findings, and conclusion.

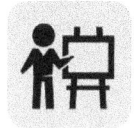

Evaluation and Analysis

Program development: Program outcomes were measured through the completion of post-sessions surveys (Appendix XX) and an end-of-program survey (Appendix XX). The post-session survey included questions regarding the overall helpfulness of the session, the session topic, the handout/activity, and the instructor; the usefulness of the content presented; and if the topic was helpful in addressing specific needs. Each question was rated on a scale of 0 (not at all), 1 (a little), 2 (moderately), and 3 (a great deal). Through the post-session surveys, participants expressed that the sessions were useful and helpful in addressing their specific needs for successful reentry.

Research-Type Project

Research question one was analyzed using descriptive data and the accompanying bar graph and percentage table.

The graph and table used highlight the level with which services are correlated to prior roles and recognition of occupations are associated with services provided by various disciplines.

Results/Findings

Evaluation/analysis: An evaluation or analysis allows for a critical assessment of the implemented strategies, data analysis, or the effectiveness of the project. The reader understands how the data or strategies were processed and interpreted.

Results/findings: Presents the findings, offering the tangible outcomes of the capstone project. Allows the reader to draw inferences and understand the implications of the project.

Conclusion: Summarizing the entirety of the project. The conclusion ties together all aspects of the project process and outcomes.

REFERENCES

American Occupational Therapy Association (2020). Occupational Therapy Practice Framework: Domain and Process – Fourth Edition. *American Journal of Occupational Therapy*, *74*(sup_2), 7412410010. https://doi.org/10.5014/ajot.2020.74S2001.

Cole, M. B. (2017). *Group Dynamics in Occupational Therapy: The Theoretical Basis and Practice Application of Group Intervention*. SLACK.

Dillon, M. B., Dillon, T. H., Griffiths, T., Prusnek, L., & Tippie, M. (2020). The Distinct Value of Occupational Therapy in Corrections: Implementation of a Life Skills Program in a County Jail. *Annals of International Occupational Therapy*, *3*(4), 185–193. https://doi.org/10.3928/24761222-20200309-01.

Fleming, R. S., & Kowalsky, M. (2021). *Survival Skills for Thesis and Dissertation Candidates*. Springer.

Jaegers, L. A., Skinner, E., Conners, B., Hayes, C., West-Bruce, S., Vaughn, M. G., Smith, D. L., & Barney, K. F. (2020). Evaluation of the Jail-Based Occupational Therapy Transition and Integration Services Program for Community Reentry. *The American Journal of Occupational Therapy*, *74*(3). https://doi.org/10.5014/ajot.2020.035287.

Salem, B. E., Kwon, J., Ekstrand, M. L., Hall, E., Turner, S. F., Faucette, M., & Slaughter, R. (2021). Transitioning into the Community: Perceptions of Barriers and Facilitators Experienced by Formerly Incarcerated, Homeless Women During Reentry – A Qualitative Study. *Community Mental Health Journal*, *57*(4), 609–621. https://doi.org/10.1007/s10597-020-00748-8.

Shelton, R. C., Lee, M., Brotzman, L. E., Wolfenden, L., Nathan, N., & Wainberg, M. L. (2020). What is Dissemination and Implementation Science?: An Introduction and Opportunities to Advance Behavioral Medicine and Public Health Globally. *International Journal of Behavioral Medicine*, *27*(1), 3–20.

15

Sustainability of Your Capstone Project

So, you have created a project that has meaning and is a contribution to the profession, your community, and/or society. Your experience has been well spent, and you now have a project that makes you feel great pride and accomplishment. But now what? What happens to the project after you have completed it? The editors of this book feel that having a sustainability plan to continue your magnificent contribution is something you should consider.

DEFINING COMMUNITY

So far you have seen the word community a lot throughout this textbook. Community is more than your neighborhood or local area. Community, from a health perspective, is defined as '. . . more than a geographic location for practice, but includes an orientation to collective health, social priorities, and different modes of service provision' (Kniepmann, 1997, p. 540) while the World Health Organization (WHO, 2010) defines community as 'groups of people that may or may not be spatially connected, but who share common interests, concerns or identities. These communities could be local, national or international, with specific or broad interests' (para. 1).

Your capstone has made a significant contribution to a community, based on the definitions above. So, let's talk briefly about how that contribution can continue, ensuring a legacy project rather than just an assignment to get through to graduate.

DEFINING SUSTAINABILITY

Healthcare project sustainability is the ability of a project to function effectively and be able to be integrated into existing resources in the community and be embraced by that same community. When interprofessional teams focus on the development of community programming, the process and outcomes of that program development require that the program be sustainable. Once a program is implemented, it is the building of community capacity that allows for sustainability to occur. Sustainability occurs when a community's needs are being met and there is ongoing evaluation of the program ensuring it adapts according to changing needs of a community. Hence, sustainability is defined as a continuous process of community partnerships that can be viewed from an individual, organizational, and community level; it is a way of thinking to build strong coalitions among community members and the external environment for the health, well-being, and quality of life of individuals and the community. No matter your site, or if your capstone project is advocacy, research, or program development, making your capstone sustainable, especially if at a site where there is no occupational therapist, can be important for 'sustaining' the visibility of your beloved profession.

The Substance Use and Mental Health Services Administration (SAMHSA, 2017) created an effective framework that can be used for any occupational therapy doctoral student, whether entry level or post-professional, to create their own sustainability plan:

1. **Assessment**: Defining the problems and issues within an organization
2. **Build Capacity**: What are all the potential resources available to assist in meeting the problems, both from a remediation standpoint and prevention of further issues?
3. **Planning**: Determining what to do and when and how to best accomplish the plan
4. **Implementation**: Putting your plan into action
5. **Evaluation**: Using your skills and knowledge in program evaluation, were the previous steps 1–4 in this list effective? If not, why not? If so, how can you build on that experience?

When using this model, consider that you might assess your progress on a continuous basis to develop a sustainability plan that is meaningful to your site.

Consider the word 'sustainability' or 'sustainable.' What does that word mean to you? (See Worksheets 15.1 and 15.2.) After you have completed Worksheets 15.1 and 15.2, share your ideas with a peer, your class, or your professor. This will give you some ideas for how you can create a sustainable project. Then write up your own narrative related to how you will sustain your own capstone. This will put into black and white how meaningful your capstone truly is.

DEFINING COMMUNITY CAPACITY

So now your capstone, along with how you view it as sustainable, has contributed to building community capacity. Your project expands on how a community can increase its ability to best serve a population! Let's define the terms 'community capacity' and 'community capacity building.'

Community capacity is the 'combined influence of a community's commitment, resources and skills that can be deployed to build on community strengths and address community problems and opportunities' (The Aspen Institute, 1996). Rogers et al. (1995) define it as 'the cultivation and use of transferable knowledge, skills, systems, and resources that affect community- and individual-level changes consistent with public health-related goals and objectives.' Your capstone is another resource and/or skill that can address those community needs and problems, and create opportunities that never existed before.

Community capacity building is 'about promoting the "capacity" of local communities to develop, implement and sustain their own solutions to problems in a way that helps them shape and exercise control over their physical, social, economic and cultural environments' (Stuart, 2014, p. 1). Similar to sustainability for capstones, sustainability is how you will sustain your program when you leave your site. Community capacity building relates your capstone project to the greater community. The overall experience is the process of developing your project with and for the organization and the community at large, making significant contributions to communities and populations while, at the same time, advocating for and expanding the reach of the profession of occupational therapy.

See Table 15.1 for some examples of how to plan for and implement sustainable projects:

Table 15.1 Examples of How to Plan for and Implement Sustainable Projects

Options	Reflect on Options You Can Do for Your Capstone
Identify methods and plan for collection of data to demonstrate program effectiveness	At the end of a program development-type project, report the qualitative, quantitative, or trend analysis to the formal leadership

Table 15.1 (Continued)

Options	Reflect on Options You Can Do for Your Capstone
How will activities and infrastructure be sustained once initial funding ends?	During the planning and implementation phase, develop policy and procedures for the institution to identify the resources to continue the capstone project. The policy statement can state the purpose of the project. The procedures identify the resources and timing that employees of the site will follow to continue the project.
Will you collect additional data that demonstrate program efficiencies and effectiveness, community advocacy, funding diversification, and collaborative partnerships that can maximize resources?	During the planning and implementation phase, explicitly plan how you could form partnership between organizations serving the same population. Develop a policy and procedure for the leadership to continue the relationships after the capstone experience ends.

Worksheet 15.1: Sustainability

Consider the word sustainable relative to each of the following. Write down your own thoughts on this:

1. One-on-one or group OT interventions

   _____

   _____

   _____

2. OT and its impact on any population

   _____

   _____

   _____

3. OT and its impact on a community

   _____

   _____

   _____

4. OT and its impact on society

   _____

   _____

   _____

Worksheet 15.2: Elements of a Sustainability Plan

Table 15.2 Elements of a Sustainability Plan

Options	Reflect on options you can do for your capstone
Identify methods and plan for collection of data to demonstrate program effectiveness (Important for newer programs)	
How will activities and infrastructure be sustained once initial funding ends? (Also important for newer programs)	
Will the target population be enlarged? (Particularly for experienced programs)	
Will you transfer best practices to other programs? (Particularly for experienced programs)	
Will you build relationships with other agencies?	
How will you build more efficient mechanisms for funding? (Such as repurposing of existing resources through improved alignment, and coordination of complementary activities and resources?)	
Will you collect additional data that demonstrate program efficiencies and effectiveness, community advocacy, funding diversification, and collaborative partnerships that can maximize resources?	
What are your plans for developing community assets through staff/volunteer training and programming?	
Do you have other plans for developing community assets?	

Source: Fazio, 2017.

REFERENCES

Fazio, L.S. (2017). *Developing Occupation-Centered Programs with the Community*. SLACK.

Kniepmann, K. (1997). Prevention of Disability and Maintenance of Health. In C. Christiansen & C. Baum (eds.), *Occupational Therapy: Enabling Function and Well-Being*. SLACK, pp. 531–555.

Rogers, T., Howard-Pitney, B., & Lee, H. (1995). An Operational Definition of Local Community Capacity for Tobacco Prevention and Education. Stanford Center for Research in Disease Prevention.

Stuart, G. (2014). Sustaining Community. Retrieved from: https://sustainingcommunity.wordpress.com/2014/03/10/ccb/.

Substance Use and Mental Health Services Administration (SAMHSA) (2017, November 26). *A Guide to SAMHSA's Strategic Prevention Framework*. Retrieved from: https://www.samhsa.gov/sites/default/files/20190620-samhsa-strategic-prevention-framework-guide.pdf.

The Aspen Institute (1996). *Measuring Community Capacity Building: A Workbook in Progress for Rural Communities*. Retrieved from: https://www.aspeninstitute.org/wp-content/uploads/files/content/docs/csg/Measuring_Community_Capactiy_Building.pdf.

World Health Organization (WHO) (2010). *7th Global Conference on Health Promotion*. Retrieved from: https://www.who.int/teams/health-promotion/enhanced-wellbeing/seventh-global-conference/community-empowerment.

16

Dissemination

You have reached the end of your capstone project and experience. It's time to show off your completed capstone project through dissemination of the outcomes of the project. The goal of dissemination is to share what you learned from the literature, development of an evidence-based project, and the capstone experience. Through dissemination, you can share your current understanding in a meaningful way to a larger community.

The capstone represents not only the conclusion of your academic journey, but also a time to share a synthesis of your knowledge, experience, and personal insight. Dissemination also provides an opportunity for students to receive feedback, enabling deeper reflection and development. By presenting or publishing, students establish themselves as active contributors to the profession of occupational therapy, fostering connections and opening doors to future opportunities. In essence, dissemination transforms an individual's academic accomplishment into a community asset that benefits both the individual and the community.

Different academic institutions require different methods of dissemination. Pick from the menu, any method of dissemination you want to pursue. Use Worksheet 16.1 to draft submissions or presentations to your targeted audience, ensuring clarity and effective communication of your key findings and implications for the future.

Menu

- **Dissemination at your academic institution**: Academic institutions host seminars, inviting faculty, peers, and community partners to review and discuss project outcomes.
- **Conference submission to OT-focused organizations**: Submit your project to relevant state and national organizations. Examples include local associations, state OT associations, AOTA, or WFOT.
- **Conference submission to non-OT-focused organizations**: Submit your project to relevant local, state, and national professional organizations. Examples include: American Congress of Rehabilitation Medicine, state rehabilitation conferences, local facilities or hospitals.
- **Academic publishing**: Submit to traditional academic journals.
- **Non-academic publishing**: Submit to publications and magazines that would share your project with relevant stakeholders.
- **Presentations at mentored practice setting**: Present your project at your mentored practice setting.
- **Presentations at a community setting**: Present your project at a location outside of your mentored practice setting.

DISSEMINATION AT YOUR ACADEMIC INSTITUTION

Your academic institution might offer an organized seminar, workshop, or poster presentation within the university or college. The audience consists primarily of faculty members, peers, fieldwork educators, and occasionally students from other departments.

- Pros: Instantaneous feedback from familiar peers, faculty, and mentors.

  o Enhances the institution's academic standing.
  o Possibilities for interprofessional collaboration with other departments on projects.

- Cons: Limited to the academic community.

  o May not reach outside of your institution.

CONFERENCE SUBMISSION TO OCCUPATIONAL THERAPY-FOCUSED ORGANIZATIONS

Various conferences occur across states, the United States (AOTA), and the world (WFOT). Each of the OT conferences focuses on the profession of occupational therapy. Submitting outcomes of your capstone project and experience expands on what is known and what is happening across the profession.

- Pros: Exposure to a larger occupational therapy audience and subject matter experts.

  o Opportunities to network.
  o Immediate input from a variety of perspectives.

- Potentially resource-intensive (e.g., registration fees, travel expenses).

  o Extremely competitive acceptance.
  o In most cases you will graduate before acceptance and presenting.

CONFERENCE SUBMISSION TO NON-OT-FOCUSED ORGANIZATIONS

You can also identify conferences outside the OT community that intersect with your capstone project. Submitting to a non-OT-focused conference will require you change the target audience to an audience with less familiarity with the profession. This includes providing additional descriptions for OT terms and providing in-depth descriptions of how the profession views health. Submission to non-OT-focused organizations is a great way to highlight the inter-disciplinary relevance of your capstone.

- Pros: Extends your capstone reach beyond the OT community, thereby gaining interdisciplinary recognition.

  o Provides opportunities for collaboration and networking with professionals from different fields.
  o Increases the student's adaptability and versatility to collaborate with other organizations.

- Cons: Extra effort (editing) is required to make the work relevant and understandable to a non-OT audience.

  o May encounter difficulties in meeting the specific requirements of a different field.

o Greater competition, as submissions are evaluated across a broader spectrum of disciplines and topics.

ACADEMIC PUBLISHING

Preparing a manuscript according to an academic journal guidelines, undergoing the peer-review process, and responding to edits to be published.

- Advantages: Permanent record of your project outcomes.

  o Enhances credibility and expands influence.
  o Can result in academic recognition and career prospects.

- Cons: The process can be lengthy and rigorous.

  o Potential for rejection.
  o In most cases, you will graduate before acceptance and publication.

NON-ACADEMIC PUBLISHING

Prepare a manuscript or article related to your capstone to send to periodicals, newspapers, industry publications, or websites. This requires making your academic content more accessible, engaging, and pertinent to a general or specific non-academic audience. Review the content published on your targeted audience and model the relevant component of your capstone to align with the publisher.

- Pros: Reaches a broader, more diverse audience outside of academia.

  o Improves public understanding of occupational therapy.
  o Creates a link between your capstone and other real-world applications.

- Cons: It may be necessary to make content modifications to focus on the mission of the targeted publisher.

  o The editorial guidelines may prioritize reader engagement over exactness.

PRESENTATIONS AT MENTORED PRACTICE SETTING

Disseminate at your mentored practice setting. Schedule and prepare to present your capstone project and share literature relevant to the setting. The presentation can be a workshop, presentation, or poster. The content can be tailored to focusing on practical applications at the setting.

- Pros:

  o Application of your capstone to the targeted setting.
  o Direct feedback from site mentors.
  o Familiarity with the staff and setting.
  o Possibilities for continued collaboration and employment.

- Cons:

  o May need to adjust the content's level of detail or language to match the audience's knowledge.
  o May not reach outside of the mentored practice setting.

PRESENTATIONS AT A COMMUNITY SETTING

Create a customized presentation, workshop, or poster for a community center, local organization, or a public interest group. The content will be edited to focus on the goals and mission of the community setting.

- Pros: Increases the level of public participation, reaching a diverse audience.
    - Can result in practical applications or collaborations with community partners.
    - Develops relationships and networking opportunities outside of the mentored practice setting.

- Cons: The content needs to be edited and presented in a manner familiar to the community setting.
    - May not reach outside of the community setting.
    - The audience has varied levels of interest and expertise.

Learning Activity 16.1: Drafting an Abstract

Writing an Abstract for Publication

An abstract is a concise summary of the content of a publication or presentation. No matter the type of dissemination type, it is common to begin with an abstract. An abstract provides a brief overview of the topic, the problem, the purpose, findings, and implications for the future. This is the initial summary that aids readers in gauging the relevance of your topic, guiding the reader's decision to pursue the material further.

Cut and paste this content from your completed work if possible:

1. In 1–2 sentences, what is the background to the problem you addressed?

    _____

    _____

2. In one sentence what was the specific problem you focused on for your capstone project?

    _____

    _____

3. In one sentence, what was the purpose of your capstone (the capstone type)?

    _____

    _____

4. In 1–2 sentences, describe what was done for your capstone.

    _____

    _____

---

5. In 1–2 sentences, what were the outcomes or findings of your capstone project?

_____

_____

6. What are the top 2–3 takeaways or implications for the future gained from your capstone?

_____

_____

7. Use the sample as a guide to draft an abstract for publication.

_____

_____

Learning Activity 16.1 Example: Drafting an Abstract

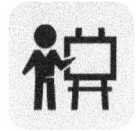

Writing an Abstract for Publication

EXAMPLE (Miguelino, 2018 – student sample)

An abstract is a concise summary of the content of a publication or presentation. No matter the type of dissemination type, it is common to begin with an abstract. An abstract provides a brief overview of the topic, the problem, the purpose, findings, and implications for the future. This is the initial summary that aids readers in gauging the relevance of your topic, guiding the reader's decision to pursue the material further.

Cut and paste this content from your completed work if possible:

1. **In 1–2 sentences, what is the background to the problem you addressed?**
   Intensive care unit (ICU) delirium is a common condition among individuals in critical care. More than 5 million patients are admitted annually to United States' (US) ICUs with a range of 45–87% incidence of delirium (Alverez et al., 2017). Delirium's negative side includes longer hospital stays; greater reliance on long term care; and motor, cognitive, and functional decline (Alverez et al., 2017; Rains & Chee et al., 2017; Tobar et al., 2017).

2. **In one sentence what was the specific problem you focused on for your capstone project?**
   The problem is individuals with ICU delirium lack evidence-based occupational therapy services to support functional outcomes, improve care coordination, and decrease role dysfunction. (Alverez et al., 2017; Barbieri et al., 2016; Brummel et al., 2014; Corcoran et al., 2017; Dinglas et al., 2013; Pozzi et al., 2017; Rains & Chee, 2017; Tobar et al., 2017; Trogrlic et al., 2015; Schweickert et al., 2009).

3. In one sentence, what was the purpose of your capstone (the capstone type)?

The purpose of this qualitative research-type capstone project is to explore interdisciplinary team perceptions of occupational therapy's role in managing delirium within the ICU setting.

4. In 1–2 sentences, describe what was done for your capstone.

Individual interviews were conducted with eight ICU staff members to discuss support, barriers, and collaboration regarding the OT's role in the ICU.

5. In 1–2 sentences, what were the outcomes or findings of your capstone project?

Three themes emerged from the interviews: 1) ICU staff address delirium through a hierarchy of needs; 2) Barriers to collaboration with OT are due to knowledge gaps, lack of teamwork, decreased motivation to learn; 3) To improve interdisciplinary knowledge, ICU staff report a need for interdisciplinary rounds or development of a delirium huddle. This research project explored the role of OT in ICU delirium management, to improve functional outcomes for individuals with ICU delirium.

6. What are the top 2–3 takeaways or implications for the future gained from your capstone?

For the future it is recommended that OT and ICU educational sessions are developed, to educate the ICU team on the role of the OT; institutional barriers are identified in order to find opportunity for culture change in the ICU; and that advocacy materials are developed to facilitate collaboration between the occupational therapy department and the ICU.

7. Draft an abstract:

Intensive care unit (ICU) delirium is a common condition among individuals in critical care. The problem is individuals with ICU delirium lack evidence-based occupational therapy services to support functional outcomes, improve care coordination, and decrease role dysfunction. (Alverez et al., 2017; Barbieri et al., 2016; Corcoran et al., 2017; Pozzi et al., 2017; Rains & Chee, 2017). The purpose of this qualitative research project was to explore interdisciplinary team perceptions of occupational therapy's role in managing delirium within the ICU setting. Individual interviews were conducted with eight ICU staff members to discuss support, barriers, and collaboration regarding the OT's role in the ICU. Three themes emerged from the interviews: 1) ICU staff address delirium through a hierarchy of needs; 2) Barriers to collaboration with OT are due to knowledge gaps, lack of teamwork, decreased motivation to learn; 3) To improve interdisciplinary knowledge, ICU staff report a need for interdisciplinary rounds or development of a delirium huddle. For the future it is recommended that OT and ICU educational sessions are developed, to educate the ICU team on the role of the OT; institutional barriers are identified in order to find opportunity for culture change in the ICU; and that advocacy materials are developed to facilitate collaboration between the occupational therapy department and the ICU.

Doctor of Occupational Therapy Program

Program to Increase Occupational Therapy Inclusion in Community Mental Health Practice

LeeAnne Bugter-vanLoon, OTDS; Subject Matter Experts: Jeffrey Sargent, OTD, OTR/L, Thomas Laster, OTD, MS, OTR/L, Doctoral Coordinators: Pamela Kasyan-Howe, OTD, OTR/L; Kristin Domville, DrOT, OTR/L; Lisa Schubert, OTD, OTR/L

BACKGROUND

Occupational therapists are qualified mental health providers, but services are often underutilized, and practitioners frequently lack recognition in their role as mental health providers (Brooks & Bannigan, 2018; D'Amico et al., 2018; Ramafikeng et al., 2020). Limited numbers of occupational therapists in the mental health community creates further difficulty understanding of the professions' role within this setting (AOTA, 2020; Estrany-Munar et al., 2021).

PROBLEM

Inadequate numbers of occupational therapists work in the community to treat individuals with mental health conditions (Brooks & Bannigan, 2018; D'Amico et al., 2018; Ramafikeng et al., 2020).

PURPOSE

To create a program to advocate for the profession of occupational therapy to increase capacity for occupational therapy practitioners in community-based mental health services.

Project Objectives:
- Develop a 2-hour workshop
- Create workshop objectives
- Advertise the workshop
- Conduct the workshop

METHODS

Setting: South Florida Community Mental Health Drop-in Center

Development and Implementation:
- Direct observational hours at a community mental health center.
- Virtual networking with community mental health organizations and constituents.
- Direct collaboration with the site to identify methods for OT funding and reimbursement in community mental health settings.
- Implementation of a 2-hour virtual workshop advocating for increased occupational therapy inclusion in community mental health.
- Program evaluation form emailed to participants via Google Forms.

Workshop content:
- OT in community health
- Community mental health services
- Guest speakers: Certified peer specialists
- Barriers that limit inclusion
- Methods for increased inclusion
- Exploration of billing and reimbursement

Inclusion Criteria:
- OT practitioners and students
- Other mental health providers
- General healthcare providers
- Mental health advocates

Theoretical Framework:
The Model of Human Occupation (MOHO)

Special thanks to Chris Yoculan, Site Supervisor and Adult Services Director, and Laura Diaz de Arce, Power-of-Peers Supervisor and Certified Peer Recovery Specialist

PROGRAM OUTCOMES

Participants: 22 total participants attended the workshop. All participants completed the program evaluation form.

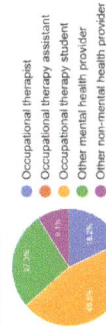

- Occupational therapist
- Occupational therapy assistant
- Occupational therapy student
- Other mental health provider
- Other non-mental health provider

Program Evaluation Results:
- Most participants (86.4%) found the workshop very easy to understand or somewhat easy to understand (9.1%).
- 100% of participants reported they found the workshop meaningful and engaging.
  - i.e., interactivity, organization, relevance
- Feedback included adding visual aids and more polls, however, most respondents indicated no changes were needed.

Additional Outcomes: Virtual networking directly with the site resulted in an opportunity to develop a pilot program directly incorporating OTs in community mental health settings.

Table 1: Program Evaluation Responses regarding increased understanding of workshop content

Questions	Responses
How effective was the workshop at increasing your understanding of OT's role in community mental health (CMH)?	Very effective (VE): 90.9% Somewhat effective (SE): 9.1%
How effective was the workshop at increasing your understanding of the barriers to OT inclusion in CMH?	VE: 100%
How effective was the workshop at increasing your understanding of methods to network for OT services within CMH?	VE: 95.5% SE: 4.5%
How effective was the workshop at increasing your understanding of methods to advocate for OT services within CMH?	VE: 95.5% SE: 4.5%
How effective was the workshop at increasing your understanding of how billing and reimbursement impact OT mental health services?	VE: 90.9% SE: 9.1%

CONCLUSION & DISCUSSION

- The virtual workshop increased participant knowledge on the roles, limitations, and opportunities for OTs in community mental health settings.
- The inclusion of multiple professions increased multi-disciplinary understanding regarding the role of OT in mental health.
- Future recommendations to include offering multiple workshops to increase attendance and response rates.

REFERENCES

- American Occupational Therapy Association. (2020). 2019 workforce & salary survey. American Occupational Therapy Association.
- Brooks, R., & Bannigan, K. (2018). Occupational therapy interventions in child and adolescent mental health: A mixed methods systematic review protocol. JBI Database of Systematic Reviews and Implementation Reports, 69). 1764-1771. https://doi.org/10.11124/JBISRIR-2017-003912
- D'Amico, M. L., Jaffe, L. E., & Gardner, J. A. (2018). Evidence for interventions to improve and maintain occupational performance and participation for people with serious mental illness: A systematic review. American Journal of Occupational Therapy, 72, 7205190020. https://doi.org/10.5014/ajot.2018.033332
- Estrany-Munar, M.F., Talavera-Valverde, M. A., Souto-Gómez, A-I., Márquez-Álvarez, L-J. & Moruno-Miralles, P. (2021). The effectiveness of community occupational therapy interventions: A scoping review. International Journal of Environmental Research and Public Health, 18, 3142. https://doi.org/10.3390/ijerph18063142
- Ramafikeng, M., Beukes, L., Hassan, A., Kohler, T., Mouton, T.L., & Petersen, S. (2020). Experiences of adults with psychiatric disabilities participating in an activity programme at a psychosocial rehabilitation centre in the Western Cape. South African Journal of Occupational Therapy, 94(2), 44-51. https://doi.org/10.17159/2310-3833/2020/vol04DoucbaB

Figure 16.1 Doctor of Occupational Therapy Screenshot

Worksheet 16.1: Dissemination

_____ Dissemination at your academic institution
_____ Conference submission to OT-focused organizations
_____ Conference submission to non-OT-focused organizations
_____ Academic publishing
_____ Non-academic publishing
_____ Presentations at mentored practice setting
_____ Presentations at a community setting

1. Identify your dissemination objectives: Do you plan to publish or present within known settings like your experiential site, or are you considering external opportunities such as a conference?

_____

_____

2. Using the identified categories of potential audiences, identify various groups who may benefit from or be interested in your capstone project.

    1

    2

    3

    4

3. Investigate what the requirements are to disseminate to your targeted audience.

    1

    2

    3

    4

4. If there are options in presentation methods, select a format. Determine if a presentation or a poster would be more efficient. Posters can convey information quickly and visually, whereas presentations are more interactive.

_____

_____

5. What format will be developed for dissemination?

_____

_____

6. Who will give you feedback on your presentation prior to the actual dissemination?

_____

_____

REFERENCES

American Occupational Therapy Association (2020). Occupational Therapy Practice Framework: Domain and Process – Fourth Edition. *American Journal of Occupational Therapy, 74*(sup_2), 7412410010. https://doi.org/10.5014/ajot.2020.74S2001.

Fleming, R. S., & Kowalsky, M. (2021). *Survival Skills for Thesis and Dissertation Candidates*. Springer.

Ho, Y. R., Chen, B. Y., & Li, C. M. (2023). Thinking More Wisely: Using the Socratic Method to Develop Critical Thinking Skills Amongst Healthcare Students. *BMC Medical Education, 23*(1), 173.

Schippers, M. C., Morisano, D., Locke, E. A., Scheepers, A. W., Latham, G. P., & de Jong, E. M. (2020). Writing about Personal Goals and Plans Regardless of Goal Type Boosts Academic Performance. *Contemporary Educational Psychology, 60*, 101823.

Shelton, R. C., Lee, M., Brotzman, L. E., Wolfenden, L., Nathan, N., & Wainberg, M. L. (2020). What is Dissemination and Implementation Science?: An Introduction and Opportunities to Advance Behavioral Medicine and Public Health Globally. *International Journal of Behavioral Medicine, 27*(1), 3–20.

Tarasova, E. N., Khatsrinova, O., Fakhretdinova, G. N., & Kaybiyaynen, A. A. (2021). Project-based Learning Activities for Engineering College Students. In *Educating Engineers for Future Industrial Revolutions: Proceedings of the 23rd International Conference on Interactive Collaborative Learning (ICL2020)*, Volume 2. Springer International Publishing, pp. 253–260.

Appendix A: Writing Guidance per Chapter

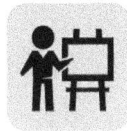

If your academic program uses the chapter system these are suggested templates to draft the introductory paragraph for each chapter.

Chapter 1

Sentence 1: The purpose of this chapter is to convey the background evidence about the problem of _____ .

    Sentences 2–3: This chapter provides a (include those that apply for your academic program background, problem, purpose, significance, and rationale for the capstone project).

    Sentence 4: The purpose and significance of a planned _____-type capstone project will be described. This chapter includes planned project objectives, rationale, and significance of the project.

Background

Paragraph 1

Describes the population. Provide statistics and definitions relevant to the population.

The Introduction Paragraph

Sentence 1: Describe the main idea of the section.

    Sentences 2–4: What you are going to be saying about the main idea.

    Last sentence – Let the reader know what will be coming in the rest of this section (big problem, little problem, link to OT, and theory).

Paragraph 2

Supporting details communicating a large/population-level problem. Provide details, facts, examples, statistics, etc. that support the main idea.

    Sentence 1: Main idea sentence/topic sentence – summarize the main point of the paragraph.

    Sentences 2–4: Supporting sentences – synthesize and support with citations information to increase the readers' depth of understanding with details about Sentence 1.

    Last sentence: Summarize the purpose of the paragraph and *transition to the next paragraph*.

Paragraphs 3–4

Supporting details communicating the piece of the problem that directly relates to the focus of the project. Provide details, facts, examples, statistics, etc. that support the main idea.

    Sentence 1: Main idea sentence/topic sentence – summarize the main point of the paragraph.

Sentences 2–4: Supporting sentences – synthesize and support with citations information to increase the readers' depth of understanding with details about Sentence 1.

Last sentence: Summarize the purpose of the paragraph and *transition to the next paragraph*.

Paragraph 5

Supporting details communicating how the problem is relevant to the profession of occupational therapy/the role of OT. Provide details, facts, examples, statistics etc. that support the main idea

Sentence 1: Main idea sentence/topic sentence – summarize the main point of the paragraph.

Sentences 2–4: Supporting sentences – synthesize and support with citations information to increase the readers' depth of understanding with details about Sentence 1.

Last sentence: Summarize the purpose of the paragraph and *transition to the next paragraph*.

Paragraph 6

Supporting details communicating the theory that will support the project. Provide details, facts, examples, statistics, etc. that support the main idea

Sentence 1: Main idea sentence/topic sentence – summarize the main point of the paragraph.

Sentences 2–4: Supporting sentences – synthesize and support with citations information to increase the readers' depth of understanding with details about Sentence 1.

Last sentence: Summarize the purpose of the paragraph.

Chapter 2

The purpose of this literature review is to provide an overview of already existing literature related to _____ (the problem). This chapter will explore common themes that presented when a thorough review of the literature was conducted. A review was conducted using _____XYZ database and _____XYZ key terms. There will be an emphasis on comparing and contrasting what the literature says about _____(themes). There is a gap between _____ X and _____Y identified and to fill this gap the purpose of this _____XYZ capstone project is to _____(purpose). The themes found in the literature include: (following headers linked directly to problem statement and background info):

Header/Theme 1

Synthesize current literature about *the population*. Provide statistics and definitions relevant to the population. Synthesize approximately 8–10 articles into approximately a 5-paragraph essay about what is currently known about the population.

Header/Theme 2

Synthesize current literature about *the problem* linked to the population. Provide details, facts, examples, statistics, etc. that support the main idea. Synthesize approximately 8–10 articles into approximately a 5-paragraph essay about what is currently known about the problem.

Header(s)/Theme(s) 3–4

Synthesize current literature about other concepts related to the problem or population in relation to the project.

Common examples of themes include: 1) Current services being provided. The gap is formed since, despite the current services being provided, the problem still exists. 2) Economic impact of the problem.

Synthesize approximately 8–10 articles into approximately a 5-paragraph essay about what is currently known about the concepts related to the problem or population in relation to the project.

Describe

Supporting details communicating the piece of the problem that directly relates to the focus of the project. Provide details, facts, examples, statistics, etc. that support the main idea.

Sentence 1: Main idea sentence/topic sentence – summarize the main point of the paragraph.

Sentences 2–4: Supporting sentences – synthesize and support with citations information to increase the readers' depth of understanding with details about Sentence 1.

Last sentence: Summarize the purpose of the paragraph and *transition to the next paragraph*.

Paragraph 5

Supporting details communicating how the problem is relevant to the profession of occupational therapy/the role of OT. Provide details, facts, examples, statistics, etc. that support the main idea

Sentence 1: Main idea sentence/topic sentence – summarize the main point of the paragraph.

Sentences 2–4: Supporting sentences – synthesize and support with citations information to increase the readers' depth of understanding with details about Sentence 1.

Last sentence: Summarize the purpose of the paragraph and *transition to the next paragraph*.

Paragraph 6

Supporting details communicating the theory that will support the project.

Provide details, facts, examples, statistics, etc. that support the main idea.

Sentence 1: Main idea sentence/topic sentence – summarize the main point of the paragraph.

Sentences 2–4: Supporting sentences – synthesize and support with citations information to increase the readers' depth of understanding with details about Sentence 1.

Last sentence: Summarize the purpose of the paragraph and *transition to the next paragraph*.

Chapter 3

Introduction

Paragraph 1

Sentence 1: The purpose of this chapter is to describe the capstone project on _ _____ .

    Sentence 2: The purpose of this project is to _____.
Sentence 3: This project addresses the problem of _____.
    Sentence 4: The project contributes to _____ by _____ (rationale).
    Sentence 5: This is significant since it _____ (fills the gap in understanding/develops a program that) _____ (significance).

Paragraph 2

Sentence 1: Project objectives are related directly to the _____-type capstone project.
    Sentence 2–3: The objectives of this project are to _____ _____ (list or summarize the objectives).
    Sentence 4: Learning objectives relate directly to developing an in-depth exposure to the _____ (population or problem) _____ _____ . Each objective will be measured by an outcome demonstrated by a deliverable.

Index

For Product Safety Concerns and Information please contact our EU
representative GPSR@taylorandfrancis.com
Taylor & Francis Verlag GmbH, Kaufingerstraße 24, 80331 München, Germany